2.07.07

W9-CAX-579

Sandie—

Allow a

passion for health &

fitness fuel a successful

journey! Carpe Diet!.

Julia

The Vice-Busting Diet

The Vice-Busting Diet

A 12-Week Plan
to Break Your Worst Food Habits
and Change Your Life Forever

JULIA GRIGGS HAVEY

with

J. Patrick Havey, D.C.

St. Martin's Press ✠ New York

www.stmartins.com

Design by Patrice Sheridan

LIBRARY OF CONGRESS CATALOGING-IN-PUBLICATION DATA

Havey, Julia Griggs.
    The vice-busting diet : a 12-week plan to break your worst food habits and change your life forever / Julia Griggs Havey with J. Patrick Havey.—1st ed.
        p. cm.
    ISBN-13: 978-0-312-34836-6
    ISBN-10: 0-312-34836-3
    1. Reducing diets.   2. Weight loss.   3. Food habits—Psychological aspects.   I. Havey, J. Patrick.   II. Title.

    RM222.2.H316 2006
    613.2'5—dc22

                                                                        2005033472

First Edition: August 2006

10   9   8   7   6   5   4   3   2   1

Dedicated to Valerie,
who accepted the vice-busting approach
and went on to lose 185 pounds—and keep it off!
Seeing how vice busting changed her life,
and the lives of thousands of others,
is wind beneath my wings!

Contents

Acknowledgments

There are many people to thank who have helped put together this book, either directly or indirectly. Whether family members who were there to encourage, or the readers whose successes continue to inspire, everyone provided a contribution. It is important to recognize everyone who has supported this effort.

St. Martin's Press has been kind enough first to consider this diet plan, and second, to believe that it would be not just a bestseller but also, most important, a best results getter. Sheila Curry Oakes, my editor at St. Martin's, worked very hard and has fine-tuned the book and clarified the message—thank you!

It is also important that I thank my agent, Linda Konner. If you want to get a book published, you really need an agent. I was fortunate enough to find Linda. I thank Linda for believing in me from day one. Public acknowledgment and recognition is one of the most important aspects of being "paid" for a job well done. Thank you, Linda.

I would also like to thank Dr. David Katz, who provided the foreword. We first met at the ABC/Time Summit on Obesity in June 2004. I am grateful for his knowledge, guidance, and for accepting me as a colleague. His knowledge and clinical experience have helped me grow. Dr. Katz, thank you for using your time and energy to support my efforts.

Huge thanks to Dr. Delia M. Garcia for her help in teaching me how important preventative care is and for showing me what steps I should take to ensure the best health and future possible.

I have to acknowledge my boss, John McGran, eDiets.com editor and "Mr. Bad Foods" himself! Seven years ago John shared my story with the eDiets readers and launched my career as the Master Motivator. He bestowed the name on me and with it came the responsibility of living up to it. I owe you more thanks than I can ever give in a lifetime. I adore you!

There are a couple more people closer to home to acknowledge. First, I'd like to thank Valerie, to whom I've dedicated this book, for all of her time and enthusiasm. I'd also like to thank Brandon, who has come into our family's life and been a real blessing for us. He also helped with the research that went into this book.

To our children, Taylor and Clark, you have put up with being without me on the occasions that I was busy helping others. It's not easy when there are moments missed, but you both have learned a great lesson, that having a purpose—one that helps others—is an essential part of life. I hope that I have made up the few times we missed spending together by being a good example for you both as you become adults. I love you and am so happy to be your mother; you are amazing people.

To my father—one journey ends and another begins. You continue to amaze me, make me laugh, and above all, make me feel loved. I pray that you and Denise enjoy your retirement in good health and humor. I can't imagine a day without you in it. Denise, thank you for the mothering; I need it more than you know and love you more than you realize for accepting me for who I am.

And to all of my extended family members and friends, I thank you for putting up with my eccentric self. All of you are such a great influence. I couldn't be luckier than to have such wonderful people in my life.

I thank **you**, the reader, for giving me (and yourself) the chance to try this whole diet thing one more time. You are ultimately the one who has to do it, but I believe you can. Enjoy the road ahead and thanks again for taking that first step of getting this book.

Finally, huge thanks go to my beloved husband, Patrick. He picks me up when I fall, supports me when I am faltering, and pushes me past where I think the goal is, making me continue to expect the best from myself and accept nothing less. He provides me with the knowledge, research, and the inspiration that I need to be able to continue helping others. Without his encouragement none of this would be a reality. There isn't a page of this book that my husband's amazing passion for health hasn't helped to create. We work together to devise solutions for improving the weight and health of others, and have done so for more than ten years. It isn't only what we do—it's who we are. We have grown together. We've laughed and cried and celebrated. Through our dreams we live, through our love we give. Patrick, I am thankful for you every day. Knowing you has made me a better person. I love you with my whole heart.

Carpe Diet,

Julia

✸ Foreword

If you could design the ideal weight loss advice, your priorities would likely include reliability, practicality, simplicity. You would want advice that makes intuitive sense, fits into your life, accommodates your family. And, if you could select your adviser, you would doubtless emphasize compassion, insight, intelligence, experience.

In other words, if you could design the ideal package of weight loss guidance, you would wind up with something remarkably like *The Vice-Busting Diet*. And if you could screen and select among candidates for the ideal weight loss adviser, you would almost certainly choose someone just like Julia Havey.

You are fortunate; no need to design advice or screen advisers. There is no one more like Julia Havey than Julia herself—so the choice of adviser is clear. And in *The Vice-Busting Diet*, Julia has dietary guidance for you that will meet your every specification, and surpass your every expectation. Julia is, in a word, terrific, and this is Julia at her best.

The advice Julia offers here is eminently sensible, definitely doable, and wonderfully empowering. It is also tried-and-true, the basis for Julia's own remarkable weight loss success. Healthy, vibrant, and 130 pounds lighter than her former self, Julia talks about weight loss—and lasting weight control—not as a hypothetical, but as a journey she knows intimately. When you follow where Julia leads, there is no risk of losing your way, because Julia has walked every step of this walk already!

Julia is clear, confident, and assertive in her guidance, as only a knowledgeable and experienced guide can be. But make no mistake: she is kind, gentle, and understanding. There is no harsh judgment, no recrimination on these pages. When Julia speaks of "vices" that need "busting" she is referring to your diet—not your character.

In this book, it is dietary vices that get the busting they deserve. What you get is protection. Vice busting is about self-defense against the obesigenic marauders of this modern world—from fast food to television. Julia is here—with gentle, unflinching strength—to help you chase them off.

By addressing diet vices, Julia is emphasizing the negatives in your diet so that she can help you emphasize the positive potential in your life. Focus on fixing what's wrong with your diet—and only what's wrong—and you wind up with a way of eating you can actually live with. This is in marked contrast to the myriad fad diets that reconstruct your eating pattern from cabbage soup to nuts, based on unsustainable exclusions, cockamamie theories, and/or cumbersome food combination schemes.

Julia correctly identifies leading contributors to the epidemic of obesity—and your personal weight control difficulties. She very insightfully inventories the leading "diet vices" in our culture. Her words ring true to me, based on nearly twenty years of counseling patients. These very habits have indeed often been a cause, or even *the* cause, of weight gain and failed attempts at lasting weight loss among my patients. Julia gets it.

She gives just as good as she gets. I like her emphasis on health, first and foremost. I like her focus on simple, unintimidating steps. I like the inclusion of family and the consideration of mental as well as physical well-being. I really like *The Vice-Busting Diet*!

Drawing on her own rich experience, Julia provides simple and compelling wisdom. She notes, for example:

> *Deprivation is not living without certain foods but living with them and being deprived of your true health and happiness!*

That's what wisdom is all about—discovering the obvious that most of us fail to see. Yes, it's obvious—but only after Julia points it out to us.

I love Julia's comments about kicking the fast-food habit:

Before I realized it, I started to look at other things that I was doing and wondering what results I could achieve by making one more positive change. My next vice to go was my frequent fast-food habit. I figured I was opting for fast food too often and I had myself convinced there were plenty of fattening foods that needed to go. I hadn't wanted to cook for the kids but I started to love French fries too! Now I actually had to cook, and it wasn't as expensive or time-consuming as I had originally believed. The kids and I actually sat down and ate together rather than them eating in the car and me eating on the sly. The benefits of that could fill a chapter in a book about raising children.

I have five children and often emphasize how vitally important it is to think *family* when thinking *diet*. Improving your relationship with your children as a by-product of losing weight is one heck of a fringe benefit!

Julia's guidance comes in simple, user-friendly increments. At every step, she accentuates the positive, from attitude to health to family. She keeps it simple. Don't reinvent your diet; just track down, round up, and chase away what's wrong with it.

The Vice-Busting Diet replaces the silly, self-defeating goal of "ideal weight right away" with success measured in actions you truly can take, outcomes you truly control. Follow in Julia's footsteps—she knows the way. Take the warm and wise advice she offers, and the empowering control she provides. Do so, and at last, your weight will take care of itself!

David L. Katz, M.D., M.P.H., F.A.C.P.M., F.A.C.P.,
director of the Yale Prevention Research Center;
medical contributor, ABC News and O, The Oprah
Magazine; author of The Flavor Point Diet

❧ Preface

Thank God for people like Julia Havey. At a time when nearly two-thirds of all Americans are overweight or obese—and the rest of the world is fast catching up—we need role models for healthy living. While that rail-thin fitness pro or stick-figure nutritionist may talk the talk, it's a former fatty like Julia who's walked the walk to wellness.

I first met Julia in 2000. She was a bright-eyed former pageant queen with a simple message: "I was unhappy. I gained a lot of weight. I found a way to turn my life around. You can too!"

I probably hired Julia more for her glowing personality than for her writing skills. But six years and 200-plus columns later, Julia remains an integral part of the eDiets family of experts, all dedicated to helping the hopeless attain a healthier lifestyle.

It's easy to lose weight. Heck, I've done it a dozen or more times. The hard part is keeping off the weight you lose. I haven't mastered that part yet. So it's comforting to have a close personal relationship with a woman who has been there, done that in the lose-weight-and-keep-it-off department.

Millions of eDiets subscribers have had access to Julia's heartfelt messaging. And from the many letters I receive, it's clear Julia has amassed a passionate following of men and women anxious to enjoy their life. Forget all that nonsense about a jolly fat person. It's not easy finding happiness when your clothes are always too tight, your health is a mess, and you need to wedge your widening bottom into an airplane or theater seat. Julia knows that pain and frustration. Not only will she never forget it, she'll never return to her out-of-control eating behavior that turned her into a sad, oversize mess.

Happy days are here again for Julia. You can hear it in her voice. You can read it in her words. After an encounter with Julia, you can't help but come away with a resolve to get in shape. If you sorely need motivation, you sorely need Julia.

So, once again, thank God for people like Julia Havey. I believe we all have a mission in life. Julia's mission is to spread the word about redemption and happy endings via proper nutrition and exercise, through ridding yourself of the food vices that landed you in trouble in the first place.

Enjoy Julia's book, then begin enjoying your life.

John McGran, editor,
eDiets.com, and "Mr. Bad Foods"

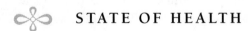 Introduction: Welcome!

Thank you for giving me the opportunity to share with you what I believe is the most effective and most logical way to lose weight and reach a level of fitness to improve your overall health. If you are like me, then you have probably purchased many diet books in the past along with other diet products, all in the hope of losing weight and keeping it off—only to be disappointed and left feeling frustrated. I'd like to say that you won't feel that way after reading and following the plan in this book. Although you've probably heard that promise before, if you take the time to go through this book and use the plan, you will find that it is "refreshingly simple," as more than a few of my clients have said. Before we begin, let's take a look at the state of health that you now find yourself in.

STATE OF HEALTH

Your *state of health,* or what is often referred to as your *overall health* or *health and fitness level,* are broad terms that encompass being overweight. You may not think you have any *symptoms* of poor health due to your extra weight, but let me assure you that having a desire to lose weight is symptom enough. If you don't realize it now, you should know that symptoms are the last thing to show up with most health problems. You don't get symptoms and then have the flu; you get the flu and a short time later you have symptoms. The same could be said for cancer—it usually takes years before symptoms show up, at which time an exam, testing, and diagnosis can be made. This is not like being overweight, where the signs become visible no matter how gradually they appear. When I use a very broad term like *poor overall health* maybe I am referring to a state of being *overweight,* which in some way may be compromising your mental, physical, social, and/or spiritual health. Instead of constantly referring to a weight problem or a weight issue, we will be looking at the big picture. This journey isn't only about weight loss; it is about YOU!

Some of the typical reasons that *you* might have for wanting to lose weight:

- To have more energy
- To feel attractive
- To be sexy again
- To think more clearly
- To find a life partner
- To wear cute clothes
- To live longer
- To achieve more goals
- To feel more confident
- To be the person you know you can be

 ## I KNOW HOW YOU FEEL

It has been more than ten years since I was morbidly obese—not a label that's easy to forget. I was 290 pounds and seriously upset about my weight and the endless attempts to lose it. I tried diet after diet, bought pill after pill, yet nothing seemed to work. Okay, maybe the diet pills would have worked better if I hadn't swallowed them with a 16-ounce regular soda. Or perhaps the Scarsdale Diet might have been effective if I hadn't rewarded myself for sticking to it all day long by eating a half gallon of ice cream at night. Ultimately, the stringent guidelines and meal plans proved too much for me to stick with for any length of time or to realize any degree of success. The pounds just kept piling on. Before I realized what was happening, I was thirty years old and weighed 290 pounds. My life was tumbling out of control; I was unhappy, overweight, and just plain miserable. Things just had to change and thankfully, they did.

I lost 130 pounds.

It was around the time that I discovered that my husband was having an affair, and I sought refuge at my parents' home. As my father was consoling me with a shoulder massage, he felt a lump at the base of my neck. Convinced that it was cancer and that I was going to die a miserable early death, I went to my doctor to receive the bad news.

To my surprise—and just as much humiliation—the diagnosis of my "cancerous" mass at the base of my neck was . . . well, just a plain *mass*. In other words, it was a mass of *fat*—a fat deposit.

On my way home, after stopping at the bakery to get a few pastries to help soothe the sting of his diagnosis, I really looked at what I was doing—eating—the very thing that was causing my fat deposit and ruining my life. I remember thinking that this really had to stop. A diet! That is what I needed. As I polished off my pastries, I vowed to start a new diet in the morning. This time, I tried some green foamy shakes. That attempt lasted about two days. Oh well, I thought the next diet would be the answer. I was too upset about the collapse of my marriage to think about dieting anyway.

Then came the straw that broke the camel's back. One night I rushed out the door after having another argument with my husband to get away and to get something to eat. I headed to the closest gas station to buy a candy bar. There I would encounter the man who would change my life. As I got out of my car, I gave my sweatshirt the obligatory tug, to pull it down so that it covered my butt and thus hid my fat from the world—or so I thought. As I walked toward the attendant's window to get my fix, a man leaning on the side of the building, drinking something out of a tattered brown paper bag and wearing clothing stained with soot and grime, loudly observed, "Girl, you got too much food in you!" He seemed to get louder each time he said it. I was beyond humiliated. Everyone, even the attendant behind the bulletproof glass window, was laughing—laughing at my fat and me. I took my candy bar and quickly retreated to the safety and quiet of my car.

Enough was enough. Too much food in me! I'll show him, I thought as I sped off. I quickly ate up my candy bar for solace.

Strangely, comfort wasn't to be found that night—not in the chocolate, not in the ice cream that I ate when I got home, and least of all, not when I took a good long look in the mirror.

I realized what the problem really was. It wasn't my husband's fault that I had gotten overweight; it wasn't my parents' fault; it wasn't the teasing; it wasn't anything that anyone else did *to* me—it was every bite of food that went in my mouth that didn't belong there.

Too much food had caused too much me!

I vowed to change. I didn't vow to diet. For the first time that I can remember, I actually realized that I had to take control.

At the time, I looked at the worst food that was present in my life that was contributing the most to my weight. One thing I knew I had "too much of" in me was ice cream. In January 1994, I said to myself that it had to go and I haven't had a bite since. You may be thinking that I've been deprived of ice cream for all this time but

Deprivation is not living without certain foods but living with them and being deprived of your true health and happiness!

I honestly didn't realize, when I first made the decision, that ice cream would *never* again be a part of my life. I simply decided not to eat it for a while so that I would lose some weight. It wasn't that difficult. The first few days I may have wanted some but I fought off the urge. After a month my clothes were looser, and I hadn't done anything other than stop eating ice cream. I realized that not eating it might just help me finally lose the weight. I was excited about the changes and that instilled a willingness to continue on without ice cream. It became a game of sorts. I wanted to see how loose my clothes would become if I continued to avoid ice cream.

The positive benefit of that one change was a perpetual wheel of motivation!

Before I realized it, I started to look at other things that I was doing and wondering what results I could achieve by making one more positive change. My next *vice* to go was my frequent fast-food habit. I figured I was opting for fast food too often and I had myself convinced there were plenty of fattening foods that needed to go. I hadn't wanted to cook for the kids but I started to love French fries too! Now I actually had to cook, and it wasn't as expensive or time-consuming as I had originally believed. The kids and I actually sat down and ate together rather than them eating in the car and me eating on the sly.

Over the next few months, other vices were busted—chocolate chip cookies and frozen icing, to name two. Even the frequent heaping of pasta with cheese needed some altering. I started to become more aware of what I was consuming that was bad, and what would be much better. I started to ask about the content or to read the label of the foods before making choices. Awareness is one of our best defenses on this journey. If you don't know the possible harm something does to your body, you may be sabotaging your effort to lose weight if you keep consuming it.

At some point after busting a few vices and losing fifteen or twenty pounds, I also started exercising. I started an aerobics class or two, and even once in a great while tried some of the muscle-strengthening machines, but was too intimidated to do much more than that. After I had lost about fifty pounds, I started to work out more often as I became comfortable and more confident in myself. I was taking step classes more often and performing some muscle-strengthening exercises as well. I started walking around the park with my children and playing with them in the playground, rather than sitting and watching while eating something as they played. In retrospect, my many hours of watching TV in the evenings was a vice that was being busted in favor of time spent exercising.

The results of my lifestyle change were evident in more ways than just the scale's measure. My clothes were getting quite loose and needed to be taken in every few weeks. My attitude was becoming more positive. Where I had once been upset at everyone and everything, suddenly everything around me seemed to be improving. My self-confidence was soaring. I no longer felt like a failure and I began to think that I was a good person with many good qualities. My time with my children was more enjoyable—we played and laughed rather than eating and watching TV. My productivity level at work was at its best, and I was proud of what I was accomplishing.

In the past, I was used to jumping on a diet and shortly thereafter falling off the diet. Then I waited until inspiration struck to get started on the next diet, only to repeat the same on-again off-again cycle. The time between diets was really the time that was wasted—you know, *waiting* for that proverbial Monday to start. The biggest difference this time was my consistency—being committed to staying on course each day. I never reverted to eating ice cream or getting back the other habits that I thought (and later *knew*) had contributed to those extra pounds. The exercise felt so good that I didn't give that up either. Even if it was only one day for the week, I went. Eventually, I stopped consuming the regular soft drinks.

As you can see, I never got into diet mode where I followed an exact eating plan and exercise routine. I simply looked at my life and decided to change one negative habit at a time. I didn't do anything too drastic and I didn't do anything that I couldn't stick with for the rest of my life. And I gave up the fairy tale that simply losing weight would solve all my problems and give me everything I wanted. Instead, I focused on taking steps to do what I could do today—because today, right now, was (and is) all we have.

I had gone through the difficulty of being overweight for many years, gaining weight and losing weight, only to yo-yo and diet myself up to 290 pounds. It wasn't healthy—I wasn't healthy. Since I've lost weight I have truly found what I believe I was meant to do in life: help others to lose weight and regain health.

 ## KEEPING IT SIMPLE

There is a common theme that I try to stick with—in my life, in this book, and with the diet plan that is provided. That common theme is *keeping it simple*. In this book, you will find plenty of information, some new ideas, and even a different approach to losing weight, but I have tried to keep the content here simple. I believe some of the contributing factors to the obesity problem today are that we have come up with too many complicated diets, have too many things going on in our lives, and have become disorganized—all at the expense of our health. Many times this complexity leads us to look for an easy way out—such as thinking a diet pill will be the answer. A diet pill or any other quick fix won't address the circumstances surrounding you or your seeming inability to lose weight. I believe I have the answer. I guarantee that you will find this approach easy to follow and that it will get results. Let's get started.

Chapter 1

How Diet Vices Have Changed
the Weight of America

Before we begin, I think we need to take time to look at what has led many of us to one of those things we do on a regular basis that can be considered a bad habit. You may know someone who smokes and refers to it as his or her one vice. Or how about someone's favorite indulgence? For example, you see someone eating some chocolate chip cookies and he or she says, somewhat apologetically, "Everyone has a vice, and this is mine."

By combining that with diet we come up with a very clear definition of a diet vice: **any habitual action that is keeping you from reaching and maintaining a healthy weight**. For example, if you eat a dozen chocolate chip cookies every day at noon, you can rest assured that cookies are your diet vice. If you drink a gallon of regular soda every day, that is *definitely* a diet vice. If you sit on the couch and are glued to the television for four hours a day, that is a diet vice. If you eat Big Macs every day, that is your diet vice. If your portion sizes are too large, that could also be considered a diet vice.

After years of helping others lose weight, I have come to the conclusion that the answer to the obesity problem in the United States lies with each of us overcoming our diet vices. This may sound oversimplified, but I truly believe, and will show you, that diet vices are probably the biggest hurdle to getting rid of the extra weight and the extra calories. It's not that we haven't had the right eating plan or known the correct food combinations or been following the proper "points" system. I don't believe that we lack the intelligence to distinguish between good and bad foods. I am convinced that we have been conditioned to believe that dieting is complicated and that we must follow a complex diet in order to lose weight.

I think what happened to me is what is happening to the entire country—we're dieting ourselves into a state of obesity. If you think about it, at one time or another you've probably tried to radically change what you eat in order to follow the recommendations of some expert's diet plan. If you are anything like I was, you couldn't stick with those radical changes and you jumped back (face-first) to the foods you ate before. That sums up how just about all of us have dieted on and off for years.

Let's be honest. I think you would agree that plenty of foods out there aren't healthy. In fact, I'm willing to bet that you not only know what foods aren't good for you but also how much of them you eat! See, I believe that we don't need an expert to tell us how to diet. I also believe I know some things about the way to live in order to achieve a healthy weight. The first thing you need to know is that identifying the diet vices in your life is the first step to gaining control of your life and your weight.

I have identified the top three diet vices that have gotten in the way of many of my clients' weight losses and have also led to the weight problems of many subscribers to eDiets.com whom I have worked with. If your vice isn't in the top three, don't worry. I will help you to identify your individual vice and show you the way to break the bad habit (or habits) that is keeping you from your weight loss goals.

TOP THREE DIET VICES

The top three major diet vices that contribute most to obesity are sugary and/or soft drinks, fast food, and television. Again and again, I've seen them as the common denominator in so many people's weight loss struggles and I've also seen studies that have borne this out.

Soft Drinks

Soft drinks and beverages that are not "diet" are by far one of the single most important items making a major contribution to the obesity epidemic. In Eric Schlosser's *Fast Food Nation* (New York: Houghton-Mifflin, 2001), he explains that "during the 1950s the typical soft-drink order at a fast-food restaurant contained about eight ounces of soda." Mr. Schlosser goes on to describe the quantity of a typical size soft drink today: "a 'large' soda at McDonald's is 32 ounces." Thirty-two ounces is exactly four times the 8-ounce size. And that large-size soda contains a whopping 310 calories. We are getting too many calories from soft drinks at fast-food restaurants. The majority of those calories come from refined sugar.

Refined Sugar—A Big Problem

According to the *American Journal of Clinical Nutrition* (1995), carbonated soft drinks "are the biggest source of *refined sugars* in the American diet." Many people drink soft drinks throughout every day. "The USDA [United States Department of Agriculture] recommends that the average person on a 2,000-calorie daily diet include *no more than* 40 grams of added sugars, which is about the amount of sugar in a 12-ounce soft drink." The ERS goes on to report that in the year 2000, each American consumed an average of 152 pounds of caloric sweeteners. These are the sweeteners you can read about on the side of any bottle or can of soda and juice drink.

The National Soft Drink Association's (NSDA) report in 2000 claims, "The average American consumed more than 53 gallons of soft drinks." That amounts to "$60 billion annually [spent] on carbonated soft drinks" according to the NSDA. You can see that about half of the 152 pounds per year of caloric sweeteners (and this is refined sugar) comes from soft drinks. In the 1950s, high-fructose corn syrup use was practically negligible, while in the year 2000 it accounted for almost 64 pounds per person (based on dry weight).

Terms like *sucrose, fructose, glucose, maltose,* and *lactose* may mean something to a scientist, but how we supposed to understand what we're putting into our mouths?

Sucrose: More commonly known as white, refined, table sugar, it comes from sugar cane, sugar beets, and sugar maples, and is the most widely used form of sugar.

Fructose: It's found naturally in fruits and honey. It can also be commercially refined from corn, sugar beets, and sugar cane. Currently, the most popular form of refined fructose is corn syrup, which is added to hundreds of products. It is about 70 percent sweeter than sucrose.

As far as nutritional benefit to our bodies, all simple sugars are empty calories—about four per gram. As for their impact upon our bodies, sucrose is the worst. It demands the production of insulin by our pancreas, causes significant fluctuation in blood-sugar levels, and robs nutrients from various stores in our bodies in order to be digested.

These figures are intended to open your eyes to the fact that soft drinks alone are contributing enough to our extra weight to make a big difference!

The negative effects of soft drink consumption go beyond too many "bad" calories. There is a physiological issue that has to do with how your body deals with or receives soft drinks. According to the *International Journal of Obesity* (June 2000) "the calories from liquids don't seem to register the same way as solid foods with the same 'bad' calories like candy." In other words, the calories from a liquid are worse than the same calories from a food. These unhealthy calories aren't processed in your body the same way as a food with the same number of calories.

Your body processes liquids much more quickly than solids, so a soft drink or high-calorie beverage won't fill you up the same way food can. Also, these types of sugars dehydrate your body.

The Caffeine Habit

An additional contributing factor to the increase in consumption of soda is caffeine. It's easy to get into the habit of having a caffeinated drink every day. It tastes good and can give you an energy boost. There may be some interesting news regarding that habit. It turns out that a study funded by the National Institute on Drug Abuse found that caffeine cannot be detected as a flavor (despite claims). Also, according to Dr. Roland Griffiths (in a Hopkins Medicine August 2000 press release), "the same is being said about caffeine that is said (and was said) about nicotine—that each is an addictive and mood-altering drug." This adds to the reason it may be so easy to become addicted to soft drinks and why there has been such an overwhelming increase in consumption over the past fifty years.

So whether it is soda or sweetened tea or juice drinks, the increased consumption of sugar (and sometime caffeine) has led to a dangerous habit that in turn has led to millions of overweight Americans.

Fast Food

Fast food and soft drinks go hand in hand and they are the one-two punch that is keeping many of us from our healthy weight goals.

According to the *U.S. Foodservice Industry,* the number of fast-food restaurants more than doubled from 1972 to 1995, and there are about a quarter of a million nationwide. This doesn't include the small cafeterias, the vending machines, gas stations, quick shops, and so on that also have various high-calorie, high-fat foods. For the purposes of this discussion, we will focus only on the fast-food restaurants.

The most common item available at a fast-food restaurant is beef, and our consumption of beef has steadily increased over the last fifty years. In the 1950s we consumed an annual average of 53 pounds of beef per person, while in the year 2000 the annual average was 65 pounds per person, and from all indications, that number continues to rise today. What goes great on a hamburger? Right—cheese! Our cheese consumption has skyrocketed in this same time period. According to the *Agricultural Fact Book*, the average "annual consumption of cheese increased 287 percent" during those fifty years. That's an annual average per person of "7.7 pounds in the fifties to a 29.8-pound average in 2000." That's enough to make a few people overweight.

What Are You Eating?

It's time to grasp the forgotten truth about many fast foods—they're high-calorie, high-fat, unhealthy foods that don't belong in your diet.

Along with the advent of fast-food restaurants we have changed other eating habits. The consumption of milk and eggs is considerably down since 1950 (*Agricultural Fact Book*). What used to be about 37 gallons of milk per person per year in the 1950s is now about 23 gallons per year (including lower fat and whole milk). In the 1950s, the consumption of eggs was 374 per person per year. In 2000 that number dropped to approximately 250 per person. So we consume a third fewer eggs than we did fifty years ago. We also eat more lean meat and drink more low-fat milk (although overall milk consumption is down). What this tells us is that despite our efforts to eat more lean meat (mostly at home) and drink low-fat milk and eat fewer eggs, the climb in obesity rates continues. How can this be? Is it all a matter of fast food? Or can it be because we are making more *unhealthy* choices than *healthy* ones? In reality it is a little of both.

We consume more bad stuff because we now have light beer, low-fat crackers, low-carb cookies, and lean meats, which seem to give us permission to have more. The fat density of foods we eat at home has decreased by about 6 percent, while the fat-density of foods we eat away from home has increased by almost 3 percent (*Agricultural Fact Book*).

Too Much Added *Fats and Oils*

One of the other facts about fast food that might interest you is the amount of oils that we're consuming. In the 1950s total added fats and oils were about 45 pounds per person per year. In the year 2000, that number was about 75 *pounds per person*. Notice that this is *added* fats and oils, not fats that occur naturally. In fact, per-person animal fat and oil consumption fell 28 percent in the twenty-five-year period before 2000 (University of Kentucky—College of Agriculture), which tells us that we just aren't getting fat from natural fat. Added fats (created in the lab) are the kinds of substances that have been tested to do the job of keeping food together, keeping it from sticking to the pan, helping it cook better . . . and, making it taste *really, really good*! You've seen the juicy hamburgers, you've seen the greasy French fries, and the tender breaded chicken pieces. Not one of those is juicy and tender from the natural fat that came with the beef or chicken. It is juicy and tender because of *what is added*.

Certain additives are being investigated for their addictive properties. These potentially keep us coming back for more and contribute to our weight problem. It makes me wonder why these additives are allowed to be sold, distributed, cooked, and consumed.

I recently saw a report about a plant in South Africa that was thought to be responsible for keeping the South African bushman from being hungry and could thus be a cure for obesity. As it turns out, it's too expensive to extract the responsible chemical from the plant and make it into a pill. I wonder if it's not the plant, but that these people aren't "hungry" because they're *not eating junk-filled diets and are used to not overeating.* After all, they live in the desert and there isn't food available on every corner. As I see it, the primary cause of obesity is the availability of unhealthy foods and/or the seeming inability to stop eating them. No plant or any other pill can address the true problem, and probably never will. We need to change the way we think about food and the way we eat.

Fast food is definitely one of the most easily identifiable *diet vices* that we have today. If we are to solve the obesity epidemic we must begin with our own efforts to get to a healthy weight. It's unfortunate but we have been feeding the wrong machine. The machine that has been fed is an industry that gets rich by selling us unhealthy items with their advertisements and with even tastier (translation: more addictive) food items. We need to start feeding *our* machines with the healthy food (and positive thoughts) that will allow us to be more productive, positive, energetic, happy, and fit.

Many fast-food companies are taking steps in the right direction, but it is not enough. When a well-intentioned customer goes into one of the bigger chains looking for a salad she will be confronted with many unhealthy options. Salad with fried chicken is shown on the menu, featured on the paper tray liners, and is the default choice. You have to specify you want the salad with grilled chicken and low-fat dressing or you will be served something with as much fat and as many calories as a huge burger. Hard to believe? Well, the popular sandwich has 560 calories and 30 grams of fat, and the crispy chicken salad with Caesar salad dressing packs 550 calories and 36 grams of fat. It's clear that "healthy" fast food isn't much better than the regular variety.

Before we move on to diet vice three, I want to remind you that even if you never eat in a fast-food restaurant you probably have a high-fat, high-calorie vice that is keeping you from losing weight. Don't worry, we'll find out what it is and get it out of your life.

Television

A vice is not only what is adding the most calories to our diet, but also what is keeping us from reaching a healthy weight. TV has emerged as a vice for many.

Did you know that the average American watches more than four hours of television per day?* What could most of us do with four hours per day in just one year? Think of the time—365 days × 4 hours = 1,460 hours. Let's say there are thirty-six weeks in a school year. If you traded in TV time for school time and were taking a full load of courses, you could have two full years of college under your belt. Television has its place, but not taking up *25 percent of your waking hours.* What could you spend four hours a day doing that you've always wanted to do, or that you dreamed of doing as a child?

According to TV-Turnoff Network, at age two we begin to develop brand loyalty, and TV watching can be addictive. As any parent knows it can be very easy to put kids in front of the television so that chores can be finished. But by doing so are we sowing the seeds for future couch potatoes? If we change our own TV habits they might spill over to the rest of the family. The point is that TV can entertain and inform but it can also suck up time that can be used for a wide range of activities.

During our hours of watching TV, we are also subjected to commercials. In 1999, more than $40 billion was spent on advertising, and the commercials we're being subjected to encourage us to eat at fast-food restaurants and indulge ourselves. So we sit doing nothing and the only motivation we get is to put high-calorie, high-fat foods in our mouths.

Ironically, television is the source of many advertisements for weight loss programs, diet pills, and so on. Would we need them if we simply turned off the TV, put down the snack, and used the time differently?

 ## TOO MUCH TIME ON OUR HANDS

Isn't our time one of our most precious commodities? By all accounts, we are putting our time in the wrong place. In fact, 49 percent of Americans said they watch too much TV when asked. I don't know if these are the 49 percent who are making the averages higher for all of us, but certainly they aren't the only ones watching TV. If

*All television statistics come from *TV-Turnoff Network,* based in Washington, D.C., whose project—*Real Vision*—is an initiative to raise awareness about television's impact on us. Visit www.tvturnoff.org for more info.

we're spending four hours in front of the TV, isn't it a pretty safe assumption that we are also snacking while we watch?

This adds up to the fact that TV has become one of the biggest diet vices in our lives. If we are sitting and essentially doing nothing, we're not burning any calories. On top of that, if we're snacking, we are adding calories to our current weight. In simple terms, we are gaining weight every day that we are in front of the TV and more weight if we're snacking while watching. No matter how small that weight gain may be, it takes only a few weeks to see a noticeable change. If you gained 1 pound for every forty hours of television, that's a pound every ten days—then after a year you would gain 36 pounds (an average of 3 pounds per month)!

With most living rooms set up to make television the focal point of each chair and sofa, we have given TV high priority in our lives, and it seems that there is always something on that will entertain us. I don't think it's the entertainment value we need to consider, but the devaluation of our creativity and our productivity—doing things that would make us feel much more gratified in the long run. Television takes away our ability to effectively communicate with our spouse, our children, our family, and friends—all in the name of entertainment. We have the highest levels of visits to psychologists and psychiatrists than ever before, as well as the highest level ever of prescription drugs for mental difficulties. Could television be contributing to the problem?

Obesity is gaining on, and ready to overtake, smoking as the leading cause of *preventable* death. That means we can prevent it through the choices that we make. With the average household having more TVs than bathrooms, it's no wonder that we have put our priorities in the wrong place. How we choose to spend our time is just as important to our health and our weight as what we choose to eat and drink.

 ## OTHER DIET VICES

Now that you have become familiar with the top three diet vices in America, and eventually worldwide, if things don't change, you may be wondering about other diet vices that may be present in your life. For instance, I received an e-mail from a woman in her late twen-

ties who told me she was overweight and wanted my help. I asked if
she could identify one thing that she was doing on a regular basis that
was contributing to her extra weight—one food, snack, drink, and so
on. She replied that she was eating doughnuts every morning and
asked, "Could that be it?" To which I replied, "You bet!"

There are certainly many other possible diet vices, especially if you
don't eat fast food, drink soft drinks, and you don't watch TV (bravo,
you've managed to avoid the main ones). If that is the case, let me be
the first to acknowledge that you are a small percentage of those who
are overweight. Nonetheless, you will most likely have other identifiable vices that are keeping you from a healthy weight.

A relatively healthy diet (remember, we're not splitting hairs here—
I'm not evaluating every last bite) can still be a problem if you are simply eating too much. The portions can be too large, for instance, if you
are having seconds with every dinner. One woman I worked with was
simply eating too much of everything. She ate double the amount that
her body needed at every course of every meal. She really wasn't eating
anything *that bad,* she just ate too much. Oddly enough she used a
small plate, but went back for seconds and thirds. I convinced her to
use a dinner plate and serve herself the correct portion the first time
and not to go back for more helpings.

Another woman I worked with was eating too much bread too often. She was eating bagels, muffins, scones, cheese bread—and con-
cluded that it was bread that was keeping her from her goals.

Many people simply eat too many calories by consuming too
much of one food group or type of food. Like the woman in the above
example who was eating doughnuts almost every morning, you may
be eating something that is unhealthy or high in calories too often—
chocolates or brownies or bagels and cream cheese. These are not un-
common examples. The key is to identify one thing that you're eating
that is the highest in calories that you do on a regular basis—that will
be *your* diet vice.

If the above examples don't describe you, take a look below.

Common food vices

(Remember, these are *vices* we're talking about *busting,* not your once or
twice a month treat.)

ice cream, cookies
chocolates, caramels
brownies, cookie dough
fudge, candy bars
pastries, scones
pizza, French fries
potato chips, crackers
desserts—cakes and pies
too much/many fried foods
bagels with cream cheese
too much cheese on too many things
buttered popcorn (with a soda?)
most high-sugar candies or "treats"
most cold cereals
most muffins
too many mints (10 calories each × 10 per day × 7 days = 700
    extra calories)
hamburgers (no matter what's on 'em)
bacon or sausage (breakfast)
pastas with cream sauce
white bread
mashed potatoes

The main point to understand here is that there really are two or three identifiable diet vices for most of us. You may be like Carol, who drank twelve soft drinks and lost 45 pounds in six months from doing nothing other than eliminating that habit (**it can be done!**); or Ralph, who broke the habit of a double cheeseburger almost every day and lost 20 pounds in three months. Or the gentleman who told me that he was watching two hours of TV each night while snacking on chips before he went to sleep, and made just *one easy change* (of not eating chips) that brought 15 pounds of weight loss in two months—without doing anything else. If you can understand what a *diet vice* is and see what the top one or two in your life are, you will be on the road to changing your weight. The first step is to identify what's getting in *your* way.

One thing I am very careful to point out is that too many diets and diet plans are designed as one size fits all. Everyone does the same thing, with possibly some minor adjustments for weight and age. The reality is that everyone has a different level of fitness, a different set of

circumstances, and different obstacles to get over. By identifying the
three top diet vices we have begun to address what appears to be approximately two-thirds or more of the source of our weight problem.
The other one-third or so comes from things other than soft drinks, fast
food, and television, and those can be handled in the same vice-busting
manner.

 ## THE RIGHT APPROACH

   Modern conveniences like the car and the computer have
made transportation and communication much easier but they have
not done anything to help us stay in shape or exert energy to accomplish our tasks or goals. Modern-day diets have not helped us to
achieve permanent weight loss either.

   You may believe you haven't lost weight in the past because you
had the wrong diet. However, I believe that practically every diet out
there can help you lose weight to some degree and for at least some period of time, *if* you follow it exactly as prescribed. Typically, however,
these types of diets are not something that can be maintained for the
long term. While they are well intentioned and can lead to weight loss,
they largely take the wrong approach. The wrong approaches have us
changing too much about our lives overnight, going one day from living in a manner that supports our excess weight to the next day when
we are to live like a superfit, health-food-eating, exercising person. Few
could make that steep slope of change with any degree of success. The
vice-busting diet plan will not only provide you with the right goals,
but the right approach, so you can lose weight and live healthy and
fit—for good. The right approach means taking one step at a time, one
that fits your current situation.

A SUMMIT FOR CHANGE

In June 2004, the Time/ABC News Summit on Obesity took place in Williamsburg, Virginia. I had the opportunity to attend and meet people from around the country—heads of marketing for food companies, TV advertisers, producers of children's TV shows, politicians from Washington, D.C., in the Department of Health and Human Services, as well as authors, doctors, researchers, and scientists—all whom have the ability to impact the health and weight of our society. The conclusion from the summit was that there are so many different things that are responsible for our current obesity epidemic, yet there is no easy solution; and that any diet will work if you stick to it, but what is missing with most people is a lifestyle change.

I came away from this event believing that it is very difficult for one person or even a handful of people to get anything done on the national level. Whether it is implementing a government policy or a new healthy menu item (just one) at a national fast-food chain, the so-called red tape that has to be gone through—from submitting the right proposal, to approval at each office, the reviews by committees—all take a lot of time, effort, and money. *Raising awareness and making a decision to take control* is the best way to influence the supply of foods and beverages being put in the supermarkets, on the menus, in the vending machines, and in our schools—all to create a healthier society.

My goal is to give you this plan, and get everyone who needs to lose weight *and wants to lose weight,* to realize that the future lies in the hands of all of us collectively. Big companies and big government will change with the demands that we set through our actions. So it is important for us to stop relying on what is an inherent belief, that companies—fast food or any food manufacturers—are looking out for our best interests; they're not. They're worried about your coming back and buying more, because they have profit margins, quarterly targets, Wall Street analysts, and shareholders all interested in more revenues. There is nothing on that list that says "By the way, it has to be healthy!" There are exceptions to the rule, but I'm talking about those that have the most influence over the greatest number of people in America.

So start by recognizing the difference between a *diet vice* and a *healthy choice*. When we take control of our own lives, and start making choices on the basis of what is good and not so good, then, and only then, can we start to make the necessary changes to win the battle that we face.

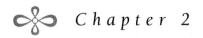 *Chapter 2*

The Positive Benefits of
Losing Weight

It is very important that you not only *know* all of the positive benefits of losing weight, but that you also focus on the *right reasons* for losing weight. A right reason could be any reason that motivates you to lose weight, but the *truly* right reasons or benefits are the ones that will keep you at a healthy weight. By setting goals, staying motivated, and achieving weight loss, you may discover additional positive benefits to your life

A healthy weight, when compared to overweight or obesity, is a body weight that is less likely to be linked with any weight-related health problems such as type 2 diabetes, heart disease, high blood pressure, high blood cholesterol, and others. A body mass index (BMI) of 18.5 up to 25 refers to a healthy weight, though not all individuals with a BMI in this range may be at a healthy level of body fat; they may have more body fat tissue and less muscle. A BMI of 25 up to 30 refers to overweight and a BMI of 30 or higher refers to obesity.

Body Mass Index can be calculated by using pounds and inches with this equation:

$$BMI = \frac{\text{weight in pounds}}{(\text{height in inches}) \times (\text{height in inches})} \times 703$$

IMPROVED ATTITUDE

A positive attitude can mean the difference between success and failure. Does that mean that a positive attitude needs to come first in order for you to succeed? No. But in order to be strong mentally, you've got to start "feeding" your mind some positive building, healthy thoughts.

I have seen obese people with a helpless or hopeless attitude. If you have 100 or more pounds to lose, it is very difficult to have an attitude of joy and happiness, but moving forward is impossible without a change in attitude. The longer you put off your goals or keep from reaching them, the more you're likely to lose hope. But as you start to take action to lose weight, through the steps recommended here, you will start to gain a different attitude about yourself. The change both in attitude and weight loss will be subtle and, like all things significant, take time. Bottom line: making even one small change that leads to weight loss can help create a positive attitude and be a confidence builder that can impact other areas of your life.

EARLY PHYSIOLOGICAL CHANGES

Your body will begin to feel better. One woman that I worked with told me on the third day of the program that she felt "weird." I was concerned until she explained that she meant she couldn't believe how much better she felt. Apparently she wasn't tired for most of the day as she normally was and felt more energetic. One of the most common positive feedbacks that I get from most people is a change in their energy level. It's not that they have an extraordinary amount of energy. They are simply experiencing closer to a normal energy level. During the first week of this plan, you will find that this may be the case for you as well.

Another positive *physiological* change that I hear is that many people get a better night's sleep. It is very possible that by the end of the first week you won't experience wild fluctuations in your sugar and energy levels, and therefore you may sleep better. In fact, a study done by doctors at Columbia University in 2004 suggested that people who got less than five hours of sleep were more prone to be overweight than those who got closer to eight hours. It's possible that overweight people have more difficulty in getting a good night's sleep. If you sleep less you may be giving yourself more time to eat. Getting enough sleep carries several benefits, including better energy levels during the day, an improved mood, fewer mistakes, and more productivity.

  ## INCREASED PRODUCTIVITY

When energy levels improve, and your confidence (attitude) improves, you will be more productive. You may find that you start getting more done in less time and therefore are more efficient. Occasionally this can create a problem: having a higher level of energy yet not having a plan for doing something productive with this new-found energy. A couple of people I've worked with have used more free time as permission to have something to eat—sometimes doing it subconsciously as a way to slow down.

Being more productive is something we often don't consider as a benefit of taking steps to get healthy, but if you start to think about what you've been putting off (sometimes for years) and avoiding, you just may be willing to give it a shot. Janice, a woman who was about 55 pounds overweight when I met her, was an artistic person who said she hadn't painted in many years because she just didn't feel like it. The truth was that she simply didn't have the energy and stopped caring about this talent of hers. Well, after about three weeks on the plan she realized that she should start painting again.

  ## MORE MOTIVATION

When my Web site posted a poll that asked, "What's the hardest part of losing weight?" the majority (about 60 percent) chose "Getting and staying motivated." It's hard to stay motivated when the plan you're doing seems like drudgery. If you've done several different diets (as surveys suggest the average dieter has), then you know it's hard to get motivated to try another diet when all the previous ones were difficult or didn't work. But it's easy to get started on the vice-busting diet plan because it takes into consideration that you probably find it difficult to get motivated and stay motivated. Once you get going and stick with the plan for a few days, you will be building up your desire to keep going—in other words, your motivation.

My twelve-year-old son, Clark, has been learning to play the guitar. The key to his staying motivated to keep learning is that he gets to play parts of songs he really likes. His teacher shows him how to play a few notes and he begins to sound like some of the music he has on compact discs. However, he also has to practice the basics so he can build on his ability to play. By learning songs he is interested in, he stays motivated to learn how to play.

If you see results, you'll increase your confidence in what you are doing and become more motivated to keep on doing it. This motivation will eventually work its way into all areas of your life—job, work, family, and relationships.

  REDUCED STRESS

If you consume too many soft drinks, high-sugar drinks, salty foods, or fatty foods, you are putting an unnecessary amount of stress on your body. This will also put more stress on you when you drive, work, spend time with family, or try to sleep. When you have toxins in your body—and let's assume when you carry extra weight that you've been putting some unhealthy calories in your body—it can make you feel stressed. When you're overweight your body works harder to function than when you're at a healthy weight and eating healthy foods. Your mind can be sluggish, your decision-making slowed, and you can even feel tense about things that should normally be handled with more ease. When you begin the first step of the vice-busting plan, you can get excited about the fact that in the next few days you may begin to notice a reduction in your stress level.

First of all, you'll start to feel better about yourself because you're taking action to lose weight. Secondly, you'll see that you won't be ingesting so many chemicals that put undue stress on your body.

 ## IMPROVED APPEARANCE

One of the most rewarding changes taking place is that you will feel more attractive. You can literally feel the few consistent changes making a difference—in the mirror and by how your clothes feel. One woman felt more confident in her appearance after only thirty days. The changes are not radical—we are not looking at setting records for the most weight lost in the least amount of time. I've had people tell me that they feel their clothes fitting looser by the third week.

An invaluable tool *to gauge your progress* is the way your clothes feel and the way you look in the mirror. But appearance shouldn't be your primary focus, because your body's changes on the inside are more important to your long-term health. Also, you may find that your weight doesn't change, even though you've lost a dress or pant size, because of an increase in muscle tone.

 ## ECONOMIC IMPROVEMENTS

As you start to experience more energy, less stress, and are being more productive, you may find that you have the opportunity to make more money. Studies from Cornell University, as reported on www.firstscience.com, show that overweight people make less money. A study of business school graduates found that men who were 20 percent or more overweight made $4,000 less a year than their thinner alumni. Regardless of how fair or discriminatory this may be, the fact is that you've got another reason to lose weight. I'm guessing that although many people may cry foul at these statistics, it may have more to do with how much they can get done. In other words, if you are healthier, have more energy, and are more productive, chances are you're going to get noticed—eventually even get a raise or a promotion.

Other economic factors will come into play as well. You will see that the time you save on missed work because of ill health will be reduced. Reports show that those who are overweight have more sick days and more missed time from work than those who are at a healthy weight. You will therefore have reduced health care costs for medications and doctor visits.

✺ PSYCHOLOGICAL IMPROVEMENTS

As you start to notice changes to your mind and your body, you will have the confidence to take more chances where you might not have before—like playing in the park or on the swings with your children, as Linda started to do after just a few weeks. Fear keeps us from engaging in activities—fear that someone will laugh at us, or the possibility of that swing breaking, which would be too humiliating to handle. Those fears will dissipate as time goes on and you can look forward to leaving them behind.

One client in her fifties didn't have the energy to take walks with her grandkids or play with them at the park. She had to walk with a cane, and her doctor told her that she had better just get used to it. After less than a year, with only a couple of simple changes in her life, she put the cane in her closet and now walks without it and plays with her grandkids. Now she uses the cane to "knock things down off the high shelves" and as a reminder of a place and time of her life that she doesn't ever want to go back to. She is motivated to make healthy choices, always.

✺ IMPROVED SOCIAL ACCEPTANCE

Unfortunately, many overweight people feel socially unacceptable or at least marginalized by society. I know I felt that my opinions didn't have the same impact as those of others who were a more normal weight. We should be valued for more than our looks, but the fact is that our appearance very often is an indication of most of the choices we've made.

Rather than focus on appearance, realize that being a healthy weight will allow you to do things that otherwise might give you trouble. You can strive to reach a level of fitness where you have fewer limitations.

Possible Benefits of Better Health and Fitness

- Show more confidence in public.
- Work more efficiently.
- Be willing to take more chances.
- Appear more attractive to the opposite sex.
- Get a better night's sleep.
- Have lower blood pressure.
- Have more energy during the day.
- Get better gas mileage (maybe!).
- Fit into theater seats more comfortably.
- Not have to purchase two airline seats.
- Walk faster.
- Have more time for yourself.
- Have increased sex drive.
- Show improved decision making.
- Wear cuter clothes.
- Save money on health care.
- Save time on health care.
- Have more time for others.
- Show more creativity.
- Set a better example for children.
- Have the ability to travel more.
- Be able to travel to higher altitudes.
- Have more potential.
- Gain more healthy years of life.
- Avoid slow death due to obesity-related illness.
- Earn a higher income.
- Live happier.
- Live longer.
- Live without regret.

SURVIVING DIFFICULT
CIRCUMSTANCES

Our health and our fitness levels won't help us avoid a natural disaster or other traumatic event, but what about how quickly we can recover? Better fitness prepares us to handle them when they do come.

There is also the issue about surviving a physical or a mental trauma. What if you need life-saving surgery that is unrelated to being overweight, and your chance of survival goes down because of your health? Is it worth making poor choices today that may put you at risk tomorrow?

When you get into a situation that you don't have control over, it can be devastating if you feel it threatens your survival. Your body responds with a **fight, fright, or flight** response. Your adrenaline starts pumping and makes you **fight** to get through it, or so **fright**ened that you don't do anything, or scared enough that you take **flight** and run away from it. How well conditioned you are—mentally and physically—will determine what your response will be. If you're fit, you might have the choice to respond in any one of these ways. But when you're out of shape, you might not have a choice.

Why not be capable, confident, and fit and healthy to the degree that you can rely on **you?**

THE ULTIMATE BENEFIT

At some point all aspects of your life start to come together: your schedule, energy level, attitude, productiveness, and efficiency—your overall health. Your mind is sharp, you feel confident, and you walk with a smile, knowing that you have developed the habits and the mind-set of someone with a high level of health and fitness. You have the energy to do what you want and to achieve your goal. You have the health to make quick decisions and be confident that they're the right ones. You will not only live a positive, healthy lifestyle, you will be a positive, healthy person! And you will have the ability to keep striving for greater goals and more successes. This is the ultimate benefit of moving toward a life with better health and fitness than you currently have. This is the goal to work toward. You are capable of achieving such a level, and it all starts with one decision and one action. Start with that one action and from there the sky is the limit.

 ## CUTTING TO THE CHASE

You will see that there will be plenty of time to enjoy weighing less, increasing your energy, and having more of whatever else it is you want; in other words, time to reach your goals and enjoy the rewards of reaching those goals.

Chapter 3

Keys to Successful Weight Loss

The surveys that we have gathered from my Web site indicate that the average dieter has been making some sort of dieting effort for about *twenty years*! The most common answer to the question "How many diet plans or products have you tried" is "Too many to count" (or something very similar). Apparently, we are willing to try just about anything, and we aren't going to stop making attempts to lose weight. If you've been on many diets before you need to know why those other attempts didn't work, and the most important aspects of losing weight regardless of the diet you are on.

DON'T TAKE ON TOO MUCH AT ONCE

The first reason that past weight loss attempts may not have worked is that you may have done too much too fast. If you have followed certain eating plans for which you have to prepare meals that are unfamiliar to you, there is a steep learning curve to get over and a major time commitment that might not fit into your schedule. It's difficult to learn an entirely new eating plan while you have a thousand other things going on. Soon you find yourself not very far from where you started, and right back to what you were doing before.

The first key is to avoid doing too much too soon. If tomorrow you try to start eating from a completely different meal plan than you have in the past, you are almost guaranteed to fail.

I think one of the reasons I've had so much failure in the past with diets is that I would try to do it all at once and thought that I had to do it perfectly or not do it at all. One thing that didn't help me was that twice I tried following the food plan for this one group and was working with a sponsor. They stress doing it all at once, and you have to do it perfectly or you've blown it and you have to go back to square one.

If you think that it's necessary to make every diet change in the first day, then think again. There is no really good reason that I can think of, or that I've read about, for changing your diet overnight. Your body needs time to adjust—so does your mind.

So avoid being overwhelmed. If you feel that you're doing too much, you are. That's not to say losing weight won't be easy, but for most people taking it in stride is the easiest way there is while still being safe.

 ## PATIENCE IS A VIRTUE

While anyone may get excited about the prospect of losing 10 pounds in a week, it is not a very smart idea because it creates an excessive amount of mental and physical stress. Although these promises may be a great selling point, we can't expect that losing any significant amount of weight in a short time period is really going to lead to lasting change. It's tempting to go for a short-term quick fix to look good for a specific occasion or event, but it's better to take care of the problem permanently so your weight won't be an issue for all the other events or holidays that come up every year.

It is much easier—and there's a higher probability that you will reach a healthy weight—if you just realize that you don't need to lose it all in a fixed amount of time. If it's three months until whatever occasion and you want to reach your goal of X amount of pounds lost by then, you need to change your mind. A certain amount of weight loss in a certain amount of time is *not* the most important part of losing weight.

If you consider how long you have been overweight, do you think it will really matter if you lose the weight in six months or ten? It will happen for you; just don't set any deadlines as to when it needs to happen.

Taking time to lose weight will also give you time to shift your mind-set toward living a healthy lifestyle. If you are anxious to hurry up and lose weight, then you are not thinking healthy for the long term. Radically changing the way you eat might not lead to lasting changes that will become part of your life.

 ## YOUR CURRENT LIFESTYLE

Most diets don't take your current lifestyle into account. We have different body types and metabolisms. We also have different types of jobs, hobbies, stresses, issues, and responsibilities. We may all experience many of the same things over a lifetime, but we are all going through our own individual trials and tribulations at any given time. It is hard to create any one eating plan that will work for everyone. Our lifestyles are a major factor in determining how easily we can handle something new in our lives. And the more easily a dietary approach adapts to our current lifestyle the more successful it will be.

 ## HOW TO CHANGE

Now that you realize why many plans may not have worked in the past (why *they* failed), it is time to look at important factors that will make this plan work. In order to lose weight, making changes is inevitable. The saying "If you want to keep getting what you've been getting, then keep doing what you're doing" holds true. Let's clearly understand the most effective way to make the necessary changes for not only losing weight but also building a permanent healthy lifestyle.

How to Lose Weight and
Develop a Healthier Lifestyle

Have a Positive Attitude. A positive attitude can spill over into positive actions and results and improve creativity, increase productivity, and even provide resources that you didn't know were available.

For any of your goals to become a reality, you must focus on all the benefits of being fit and living a healthy lifestyle before you begin to take action. Doing so on a regular basis will provide more strength, motivation, and desire to succeed.

Positive attitude is more than just saying you can do it; it is truly believing that you can, and having a conviction that you will—no matter what.

Take One Step at a Time. When you take the time to do one thing at a time, you will improve the quality of each task.

Trying to make too many changes in your life in a short period will overwhelm your brain, and you'll quickly go back to old patterns of behavior.

I learned firsthand; it was only after I gave up the demands of many diet plans and radical diet preparations that I realized I needed to choose one thing that I could change. But by focusing on doing that one thing, I was happy to see something getting done and a change being made. *You can achieve a major goal by looking at the smallest achievable goals that you can accomplish.*

Focus on Actions. Actions are the daily tasks you can complete while working toward your ultimate goal. I'll cover this in more depth later, but for now it is important that you have the actions you need to take (for your entire day) written down consistently each day. That way you can see what to do and at the end of the day you will know what got done. If you didn't complete everything, then you schedule it for tomorrow. The focus should be on *your* schedule.

Remember, you can't change your weight today without *first changing what you do.*

You may think that the scale is a way to keep score—it's not! Okay, it may be a way to note your progress, but it is the *least important way.* If the scale were the best way to keep track of your progress, you could fool everyone and use unhealthy and dangerous ways to lose weight—i.e., bulimia, drugs, surgery, starvation—and those aren't healthy actions. Think about only working on developing *positive habits*. And there are two parts to that: positive, which means it must be healthy; and habits, which means you want your actions to become permanent.

Putting your focus on only your actions, not your weight, and only on *one action at a time* is one of the aspects of this program that differentiates it from any other diet plan.

Don't Tell Anyone You're on a Diet. What is the first thing all of us do when we start a new diet? We are excited about what's to come—the new supplement, new foods, or new exercise program. Usually the excitement wears off after the first few days and we are then left with a feeling of defeat.

According to surveys I've conducted on my Web site, the average number of years that respondents have been dieting is almost twenty. That means that for most of our adult life, those who responded have been trying to diet or always thinking about dieting, or doing something to lose a pound. This seems to be a tremendous trend for those of us who have seen a weight of 50 or more pounds beyond an ideal weight. The more we gain the more we become consumed with what we're eating and how we feel. We then let our mood dictate whether or not we should eat. What we eat and how much of it influences our mood as well, and so the cycle continues. After being so consumed with the weight over the years, it is very easy to give a tremendous amount of attention to a new diet, plan, or program—even if it is just using a supplement. This can make it very difficult because you feel anxious to get results, which may lead to weighing-in every day. You can't do that—you shouldn't do that. This is another reason that you must almost forget the fact that you're making changes; just be patient and focus on what you need to get done for the day.

   ## GETTING OVER THE HUMP

When we decide to take up any significant project, goal, or lifestyle change we may hit some resistance after our first energized burst of commitment. We'll have to push ourselves a little harder to get beyond the resistance and to the point when the changes we are making become the way we live our lives.

The key to getting over *the hump* is persistence and patience. You can't speed up time, and you also must be persistent with your initial actions. That means not letting excuses get in the way of doing what you need to do (and don't worry, it's not that hard). After putting in the effort consistently for about twenty-one days, the effort gets easier. Now I'm going to give you a twenty-one-day plan that works.

Chapter 4

The Vice-Busting Diet Plan: Getting Started Weeks 1–3

 MY GUARANTEE TO YOU

I want to give you at least a guarantee of sorts so you know that your time and dollars are not just an investment in this book. I want you to make an honest effort to follow this plan for the full twelve weeks. If you need support and encouragement I invite you to visit my Web site. Someone who has succeeded in using this plan will try to answer your questions or help you with any challenges or problems. I guarantee that we will be here to help you keep moving forward. So don't be afraid to see how I and others can be of help to you and support your efforts. Reach out; you are not alone! Go here: www.ViceBusting.com.

YOUR PROMISE

Now that I've made a promise of sorts to you, I want you to make a promise—not to me, but to yourself. You have to promise that you will keep an open mind. I know it sounds easy to say, but trust me that things are going to be kept simple. Change is one of the hardest things we face, and it gets harder as we get older. We get comfortable in our routines, habits, and schedules when we don't need to think about them too much. That's why we like them—the more we stick to doing what we do, the easier it gets. So part of your promise is knowing that in the hours, days, weeks, and months to come, there will be change in your life. Stick with these simple changes—the results are certain to surprise you.

> *I promise to bust my vices, one at a time. I promise to say my affirmations daily. I promise to forgive myself for past "dieting failures" and realize that they have no bearing on my future. I promise to take inventory of all of my positive and wonderful qualities and think of them often, especially when I am tempted by any of my vices. I promise to give myself the time that I need to change a lifetime of unhealthy habits and not set unrealistic expectations.*

Sign: _____ Date: _____

As you take these first few steps, let's begin by understanding one of the other tools you have that can make or break your success: your mind. Your thinking has to change at the same pace as your physical changes—gradually. Making too many changes in your beliefs (or trying to) will be overwhelming and cause you to throw in the towel. It is different from taking action to reduce your weight—there is a higher probability of success when the change is gradual.

The same holds true for the mind. Your thinking about such things and your habits and beliefs—in regard to soft drinks, fast food, or television—may take time to change. I'm giving you the information, the statistics, and the plan that has worked for so many, and letting you determine, based on what you do and who you are, whether the same applies to you.

AFFIRMATIONS FOR A POSITIVE ATTITUDE

One of the most influential factors to your success is your attitude. There really is no substitute for a positive attitude. An athlete having all the talent in the world won't change a coach's mind if that athlete is hostile, uncooperative, and not a team player. In order to build a positive attitude, there is one action that stands out as being specifically intended for your mental strength. That action is the use of **positive affirmations.**

There have been many books that cover the subject of positive affirmations and positive thinking from people like Dr. Norman Vincent Peale, Zig Ziglar, Mark Victor Hansen, Tony Robbins, and Napoleon Hill. All of them repeat the same basic principle: *in order to improve your attitude, you've got to think positively more often.* I recommend using positive affirmations on a daily basis. Read them first thing in the morning and last thing before going to bed. It will take you approximately thirty seconds each day (total)—that's it! All in the name of being happy, confident, excited, passionate, and (more) enthusiastic about life! I suggest the following affirmations—of course, there's always the option of coming up with some on your own or from an expert in this field. (I would *highly* recommend *The Power of the Subconscious Mind* by Dr. Joseph Murphy.)

 Daily Positive Affirmation

I have unlimited confidence in my abilities and myself. I am thankful for the endless opportunities that each day provides. I welcome optimal health into my life!

If you've never used positive affirmations, you may think there's no real point in them. Please proceed with an open and willing mind. Eventually, you will begin to be stronger in your beliefs and your confidence—and your overall health. By saying the affirmations you will be programming your subconscious mind to believe that your conscious decisions should be directed toward health. This little bit of added positive thinking each day will build your brain the way lifting weights builds muscle. Reaching a major goal requires overcoming doubt, negative thinking, ridicule, and temptation—most of the time from your own mind. Do this every day and you will have that extra strength you'll need to overcome those barriers to a permanently healthy and fit lifestyle.

As you embark on the plan presented in the following pages, remember that you're not going to do it all in one day. Please feel free to read ahead and see what the next weeks have in store for you but when you come to the last page, go back and start from Day 1 and do day to day, week to week.

You should have a good idea by now of the main obstacles that are keeping you from a healthy weight. These are the things that you need to get control over. That is what must be addressed and even eliminated. Remember, the key to success isn't a matter of following the right eating plan; it is a matter of *getting rid of the wrong eating plan.*

WEEK 1: BUSTING SOFT DRINKS

Day 1

Action: Add water.

Let's first address what can be substituted for soft drinks or any other high-sugar/high-calorie drink that you may be consuming on a regular basis. Your first action—one that will develop into a healthy habit and will change your life dramatically over time is **making water an important part of your everyday life.**

Substituting water for high-calorie liquids (and their refined sugars) will result in zero calories, adequate hydration, optimal body functions, and better focusing. You'll replace toxins with clean and healthy fluids, sluggishness with more energy, expensive drinks with inexpensive or free water. And the time you spend buying unhealthy drinks can be better utilized.

 ## ADEQUATE INTAKE OF WATER

I'm willing to bet you aren't getting enough water. There are many benefits to making water an important part of your everyday life, including the fact that it acts as an *appetite suppressant.* The first step is increasing your intake of water to *an adequate level* each day.

According to Dr. Batmanghelidj, author of *Your Body's Many Cries for Water,* water can act as a fairly effective appetite suppressant. Dr. B. recommends drinking two 8-ounce glasses of water about twenty to thirty minutes before sitting down to any meal. This will provide enough time for the water to settle and give you a partially satiated feeling. Then you won't feel the need to rush to eat, and when you do, you won't feel the need to eat as much. You should also know that sometimes the feeling you have of being hungry is not a hunger pang at all, but your body's desire for water. Therefore, if you try drinking water when you feel hungry, you will either suppress your appetite or quench your thirst. In either case you won't feel the need to fill up on food.

Water's Health Benefits

Water has many other important functions:

- Carries nutrients in the body.
- Lubricates joints.
- Helps regulate body temperature.
- Cleanses the body of waste products.
- Excretes wastes through urine.
- Acts as a solvent to dissolve and carry many substances (minerals, proteins, carbohydrates, and vitamins).

If you have joint problems, it's possible that you have not been properly hydrated for several months—or years. Some people who suffer with arthritis may have heightened symptoms due to a lack of water consumption.

It is suggested that we have undigested waste in our colons after years of use (or abuse). With our consumption of so many fried, oily, and fatty foods it's no wonder that without adequate water there would be accumulated waste lodged in our digestive system. Water keeps us hydrated and helps all of our systems run smoothly.

❦ BUSTING UNHEALTHY BEVERAGES

By drinking the proper amount of water each day you'll have no choice but to get rid of those unhealthy, high-calorie, high-sugar drinks. You get two for one—giving your body an adequate supply of what's been missing from your diet (water) and getting rid of what your body is not keen at all on accepting (high-calorie beverages). Soda isn't the only beverage that is loaded with sugar. See what you're frequently drinking from the following list:

Capri Sun—most varieties
Coke, Pepsi
Dr Pepper
root beer

Hawaiian punch (and most types of punch)
Seven-Up, Sprite, Mountain Dew
Gatorade, Red Bull, and other "energy" drinks
milk shakes, Slurpees, high-sugar smoothies
lemonade
Snapple
iced tea, sweetened
apple juice
orange juice or grape juice from concentrate
chocolate milk, whole milk
café mocha, café caramel machiatto (and most gourmet coffee
    drinks, hot or cold)
wine, beer, alcohol (too much)

In fact, any drink that keeps you from consuming plain water as 90 percent of your total liquid intake on a daily basis would fit on this list.

If your current beverage intake consists of these high-sugar drinks, by making the effort to get more water into your diet you will have to choose water over these types of drinks.

Getting Started

Get yourself a few water bottles with the pop-up cap (makes it easier to drink). Those are at least 16 ounces. Buy a 12-pack if you can. Today and from this day forward, I want you to always have one of those bottles with you when you leave the house. Don't worry about anything else right now—not what you're eating or if you're getting the right exercise—we'll get to all that. Right now, drinking water is the most important action in your life related to your body's state of health and weight. The only focus you need to have today is being sure you have adequate stocks of water bottles and a water bottle within reach at all times in the bedroom, at your office, wherever.

 Daily Positive Affirmation

I have unlimited confidence in my abilities and myself. I am thankful for the endless opportunities that each day provides. I welcome optimal health into my life!

Day 2

Action: Build the habit of having water with you at all times.

Now that you've taken the all-important first step to break your first diet vice by replacing it with much-needed water, it is important that you estimate how much an adequate amount is for you. While everyone's needs are different, a general estimate of how much water we should aim to consume is very easily determined by this formula:

Your body weight (in pounds) ÷ 2 = targeted ounces of water per day

Dr. Batmanghelidj explains that half of your body weight in ounces is a good starting point for determining what you need each day. For my 155-pound body, I need approximately 75 to 80 ounces per day. Many of you may not like water. In my experience, if you are one of those people, it is possible that you have been consuming too many high-sugar, high-calorie beverages (i.e., soft drinks) for too long. So start slowly; try one glass of water in place of one soda. Your taste for water may take time to develop but it will be well worth the effort.

 CREATING A POSITIVE HABIT

If you're concerned that you'll never be able to drink the recommended amount of water for your weight, don't worry about that right now. Again, focus on getting more water than you did yesterday, and shoot to reach a certain number, like 64 ounces per day, before worrying about drinking what's recommended. If you get halfway to that number, I'm sure you will be feeling the benefits enough at that point to either increase the amount you're drinking, or continue to get as much as you are now. Work on achieving that 64-ounce per day mark; then see how great you feel and whether you should/can go on.

The most important part of this action is **getting in the habit** of having your water bottle within reach just about everywhere you go and drinking from it regularly.

Daily Positive Affirmation
I have unlimited confidence in my abilities and myself. I am
thankful for the endless opportunities that each day provides.
I welcome optimal health into my life!

DAY 3

Action: Continue to build the habit of having water with you and
drinking it often.

Often when we start something new, we stop shortly after we've begun. You may find that you're very excited about the possibilities of
making some progress and succeeding with this program and step-by-
step approach. At times that can lead to wanting to skip ahead and do
too much too soon. Or it can lead to slacking off because you realize
the simplicity of such a plan, which makes you believe that you can do
it anytime. One way to keep yourself on track is to be sure you have a
visual idea of what your goal is.

VISUALIZING YOUR HEALTH AND FITNESS GOALS

I recommend visualizing what you would like to do when
you reach a better health and fitness level. You probably have a general
idea about wanting to look better or have more energy. If you can define your goals or dreams clearly you'll have a better chance of achieving them. For instance, why do you want to look better? Is it to be more
attractive to your spouse, boyfriend, or girlfriend? Or if you don't have
anyone, is it to attract one of those three? Or maybe you feel that you
would have more attention and respect from those around you for
something more than your compassionate heart. And what about having more energy? If you did, would you work harder, play harder, travel
more, sleep less? What more could you gain from work—and what
would that do for you or someone else? What type of playing do you

want to do that you aren't doing now? Playing with your children or grandchildren? Maybe you want to play tennis or racquetball or go skiing. How about climbing Mount Everest? Would you travel to Europe, Australia, or the North Pole?

There are endless possibilities and a finite amount of time. Imagining what's possible can serve as motivation to stay on track. Visualize what you would be doing with more energy, how you might look different, what types of clothes you might buy, or even how you would feel when you wake up in the morning. The key is to find what will motivate you and then ask yourself, "Why do I want that?" or "What would I do if . . . ?" Not only will you discover some of the things you want but you may just realize that you don't have to wait until you've lost weight to do many of them—you've been letting the extra weight be an excuse for *not* doing them.

Start creating a vision of things to come—not just how you'll look, but what you'll do and how you'll feel. Picture yourself doing what it is you do or would like to do, whom you'll be doing it with, and where you'll be doing it. You don't need to have the perfect body and perfect weight to start visualizing the person, the things, and the events you want in your life.

    ## TAKING INVENTORY

One of the things I want you to do today is to take a detailed inventory of the soft drinks, sodas, juices, or other high-sugar beverages you have around the house that need to be eliminated. I encourage you to throw out all of them. (If you have some in a cabinet or bar that are used in mixed drinks you may keep those.) Otherwise, toss those empty calories. Think of it as *throwing bad health away*. If the waste troubles you, take what you have to a shelter or food bank.

Start with tossing out the soft drinks and then slowly cut down your juice consumption. As soon as you're done with the juices you have, buy no more. If you want a little juice make it orange, apple, grapefruit, or something similar but **not from concentrate**.

Remember, in place of the soda or juice, drink water.

One last word concerning alcohol: beers and wines are high in sugars, and the calories are just as many as in typical sweetened drinks and should be treated the same way.

 Daily Positive Affirmation
I have unlimited confidence in my abilities and myself. I am thankful for the endless opportunities that each day provides. I welcome optimal health into my life!

DAY 4

Action: Keep building the habit of having a bottle of water with you or being within reach of water at all times, and drink plenty of it during the day. Choose water over any other beverage.

Have you found it difficult to break the habit of those high-calorie drinks? Take a moment to relax and think about your body, how it looks, how it feels, and what condition your insides may be in. Know that you are making changes that will have a beneficial effect on your body.

We often take for granted things that we do just because they are expected of us, such as brushing our teeth, bathing, paying taxes, and so on. Too often when it comes to our weight we have to be dragged, kicking and screaming, to do what is good for us. Our resistance is borne out of being told to radically change our eating habits or lifestyle or to conform to expensive prepaid food or supplements. Water is essentially free and drinking enough of it is one of the most simple and effective steps you can take toward better health. So continue to make sure you have water within reach and drink it often.

BREAKING ADDICTIONS

As you make the transition to drinking more water, you may discover that soft drinks and other sweetened drinks are an addiction. That rush of sugar or caffeine was a hook that kept you consuming the same beverage throughout the day. Watch for bad habits that have led to addictions. Do you stop for gas and also go in to grab a soft drink while you're on your way to work or coming home? Is it possible that you've let the soda machine down the hall become an addiction when you were looking for a break from your desk? Many people that I talk with have gotten into these very unhealthy habits without even realizing. We're using the same principle to get you to incorporate a healthy habit of water into your daily life.

CHANGING YOUR MIND-SET

For a long time losing weight has been thought of as a one-dimensional process. Diet gurus discuss some variation of what to eat, how to eat, when to eat, and what exercises to do and how and when to do them so that theirs seems like a complete plan. What's been left out of the equation is YOU. Diets do not include every aspect of *your* life when considering what needs to be done to lose weight and be healthy and fit. An aspect of you that must be taken into account is your mind.

You must change your mind-set about weight loss, fitness, and health. Each decision you make can and will ultimately affect your health. The job you take, the number of children you have, the amount of water you drink, how much fatty foods you eat, how fast you drive your car—all can and do have an impact on your health: your stress level, your energy level, and, yes, your weight. Therefore, it is important that you start to view everything you do as having some impact on your health. This is part of the process that involves changing not only how you view losing weight, but your overall health. When you change your mind-set from one of "I need to lose weight" to one of "I need to get healthy and fit," then you will be taking a strong step in the direction of a *lifestyle of health and fitness*.

Don't think that you can be a part-time water drinker until you're at the office or until you're with family during the holidays. No one can succeed long term if he or she is making healthy choices only part time. **Your health is a full-time job.** It doesn't mean that you always have to be doing something that improves your health, but it does mean that when you aren't, you can't be doing something that is unhealthy. When you're not drinking water (or later, eating healthfully and exercising) you can't be someone else who eats doughnuts and fast food and drinks soda.

Health is an all-or-nothing game. If you want to live by practicing moderation, fine. But wait until you have mastered the vice-busting diet plan before you begin to practice moderation. Otherwise, you'll never know if you have control over those foods and beverages that may just have control over you right now. Gain control now, and later you can decide if you want to reintroduce these (and other items) back into your life.

This plan takes an easy approach. But in order to be successful, in control, and healthy, you must build on each step so that there are more times during the day that you are eating and acting healthy than not healthy. Ideally, you'd like to get to the point where every dimension of your life is healthy so that you're living healthy everywhere and all the time.

 Daily Positive Affirmation

I have unlimited confidence in my abilities and myself. I am thankful for the endless opportunities that each day provides. I welcome optimal health into my life!

DAY 5

Action: Keep building the habit of having a bottle of water with you or being within reach of water at all times, and drink plenty of it during the day. Choose water over any other beverage.

As you move on today and continue to cleanse your body with more water and fewer not-so-healthy beverages, you should begin to feel more energy and quite possibly as though you've lost some weight. It is amazing what results you can achieve with this one simple action. Like anything, though, it takes time. Your body will begin to do what it's meant to do: be an efficient, functioning, healthy, and energetic system.

OVERCOMING MENTAL BLOCKS

You have many things to overcome as you begin the journey to better health and fitness. The first is probably overcoming the doubts you may have about this plan. Because this plan is *about you* and what *you* need to do to lose weight and achieve better health, the first mental block to overcome starts with not believing that with this plan you are capable of achieving the weight loss you desire. (If you're like I was when I weighed 130 pounds more than now, you are in a hurry to believe that the latest fad diet is the thing to do—not only because it will work, but also because everyone is doing it so it must work!) But beyond that there exist many other mental blocks that I've encountered in my own weight loss attempts and in those of others too.

One block has to do with belief in yourself. One of the reasons it is very helpful to do the visualization exercise we talked about on Day 3 is so that you can start seeing yourself as a different person—one without the extra weight. Perhaps because of so many diet failures, you don't really believe that you'll attain a more desirable weight than you have now. You can do the latest diets, and buy all kinds of products with crazy claims, but I think subconsciously you believe that where you are now is where you'll be three months from now and possibly three years from now. Change requires moving away from the direction you've been heading in, but more importantly it requires that you start to see yourself in a different place weeks and months from now. Jumping on the latest diet doesn't make you someone who is always trying to lose weight and just can't seem to succeed. It makes you someone who is always dieting.

You must first decide that you truly want to be healthier and fitter than you are now. By making the decision to do the steps in this vice-busting plan, you will gain the strength, the desire, the motivation, and the determination that you need to succeed.

Another common mental block has to do with something entirely different that many people aren't even aware of, and it's called self-sabotage or deliberate acts of failure. Many things in your past, recent or distant, may be keeping you from succeeding and may fuel the desire to fail. If you have had one or more emotional experiences that have left you feeling angry, depressed, resentful, or spiteful, it can translate into a desire to fail.

A further mental block has to do with relatives who are also overweight. A young woman whom I helped at the request of her mother seemed to want to lose weight very badly as she was becoming an adult. She felt as though she had missed out on some very fun years and she didn't want to let her twenties turn out the same way. After a few days of helping her, I discovered something about her mother that changed what we needed to do. It turned out that her mother was almost 100 pounds overweight, just like her daughter. In our discussion, we both learned that she (the daughter) was reluctant to lose weight because she was fearful of her mother's resenting her. They were very close. In fact, her mother also did not want to lose weight because she felt that she would lose that connection with her daughter. The bottom line was that both mother and daughter needed to take steps to lose weight together and to know that they were both doing it for the right reasons.

The point here is not to let your past, others' opinions, or a family situation get in the way of your achieving weight loss and better health. More importantly, take time to reflect on what may be causing mental blocks or barriers that you aren't even aware of, so you can handle them.

Today, work on being mentally strong and prepared for the road that lies ahead. You may find that emotional reasons have been inhibiting your efforts. It is important to try to identify them clearly and bring them out in the open. The first step to moving past emotional issues is being able to look at them for what they are, discussing them with the person involved, or discussing them with someone who understands and can relate. The chats on my Web site are great for this kind of thing (www.vicebusting.com), or consider seeking therapy if the issues cause you great concern. Also, be sure that you have your bottle of water with you and are getting plenty of water each day.

 Daily Positive Affirmation

I have unlimited confidence in my abilities and myself. I am thankful for the endless opportunities that each day provides. I welcome optimal health into my life!

DAY 6

Action: Keep building the habit of having a bottle of water with you or being within reach of water at all times, and drink plenty of it during the day. Choose water over any other beverage.

As you make progress toward eliminating soft drinks and other high-calorie beverages, let's make a quick assessment of how you are feeling. Most of the people who have shared their progress with me up to this point have reported many positive results—even after five days!

Melinda first contacted me about wanting to lose more than 100 pounds. It took Melinda almost three weeks to get to the level of drinking water that was good for her body, but she had two positive effects from this first step. Even after only five days she noticed that she actually had more energy and felt much less tired than when she was drinking soda. The second positive benefit was a decrease in her appetite. She didn't feel like snacking in her car as much as she had before she switched to water.

Increasing Your Commitment

Like anything that has positive benefits, creating a commitment to drinking plenty of water each day is important. You can take another step to making water important to you and those around you in several ways. The first is to be sure that you have plenty of water bottles available. You can choose any brand that has the type of bottle you like. I suggest the sippy-straw pop-top type for ease of use. You can also buy cases of water in bulk so you have full bottles around when you need to just grab one and go. However, this can be expensive, because you'll find yourself buying at least a case or two a week. I suggest buying a case of water bottles and also getting a water pitcher with a built-in filter. You can always have filtered water on hand (in the refrigerator) at home. Or get a reusable water bottle and use filtered water. You can install a filtration system on your sink, but I've found that it's much easier, quicker, cheaper, and there is less potential for leaks and messes, by using the water pitcher with the changeable filter. Every two months or so you'll change the filter and every month get a new case of water.

If you get in the habit and continue to build on that habit and build on the commitment, you will find that not only will your weight and your health improve, but that you'll be drinking water without thinking.

SIMPLIFYING YOUR LIFE

One of the best things that I've realized about making water my number one beverage—in addition to losing weight, feeling more energy, busting a diet vice, having healthier-looking skin and hair, and overall better health—is how this one step has really simplified my life. When everything in your diet begins with water, you really get a sense of what is important. For instance, when you're feeling hungry and you're in the middle of doing something—maybe at work or with the kids or with your spouse—you don't have to think about eating and what to eat and where. The first thing you do is just reach for your water bottle and take a swig because you know that you may be thirsty. Another point is that even if you need to eat, you've just helped to defer your appetite until a time and a place that is more convenient to sit down and have a healthy meal or snack. How great is it that you get to continue on with what you're doing, whom you're with, and where you are just because you have water?

Remember, drinking water is the most important and most significant action in this plan, which is why it is first. It is really the easiest action as well. So continue to build on the habit of drinking water and focus on making it 90 percent of your total beverage intake, as well as striving to reach the right amount for you each day.

 Daily Positive Affirmation
I have unlimited confidence in my abilities and myself. I am thankful for the endless opportunities that each day provides. I welcome optimal health into my life!

DAY 7

Action: Keep building the habit of having a bottle of water with you or being within reach of water at all times, and drink plenty of it during the day. Choose water over any other beverage.

❧ WEEK 1 REVIEW

One way to determine the success of any diet program could be by the scale. But the numbers on the scale are not the only measure of success. In fact, if you never look at a scale again I would say that's fine. The best measure of how well you are doing is for you to evaluate two things.

The first is your feelings. How have you felt during the past week, and how do you feel now? Are you feeling more energy, less sluggishness? Are you getting a better night's sleep? Do you have more energy at work? Are you more productive? You don't need to go into too much detail after one week, but get a general idea of how things went overall. You will find some answers about the progress you've made, but you'll also be conditioning your mind to recognize when you do feel better, lighter, and have more energy during the days ahead. Following are some questions you might ask:

How do I feel about my progress up to this point?
How does my body feel now compared to when I started?
Can I do more to improve upon what I have done so far?
Is this something I think I can do for the rest of my life?

The second thing to evaluate is your actions. Look at the past week and ask yourself how well you adhered to what was asked of you. You should be more concerned (and rightfully so) about **what you have done and are doing** with your time than you should be about what the scale says.

Look over the past few days and give an honest answer about whether you made a valiant effort to drink more water and if you have made progress since Day 1. If you can answer with a firm yes then I say, "Well done." If you can't answer with a firm yes and believe you slacked a bit or went nowhere at all, don't worry; you can renew your commitment to make that change.

Cheryl, from Texas, has twin daughters. Like her, they were both overweight and loved their soft drinks. I got Cheryl to reluctantly agree to try the vice-busting diet and she worked on replacing her five big-gulp-a-day soft drink habit. However, her daughters busted their soft drink habit as well. They had limited access to soft drinks because their mom stopped swinging by the food mart five times a day to buy hers. Over an eight-month period, Cheryl lost 75 pounds, and her daughters each lost about 25. She also saved a lot of money, time, and possibly prevented future health problems by just making this one change. She also found a better-paying job and soon after was dating a nice man. Did all of these changes come just from busting soft drinks? There were certainly other healthy changes made along her journey, but they all started with the first step of eliminating soft drinks and creating a strong foundation from that one success. One success can ripple into other areas and create positive results.

Carol was not diet deprived. She had tried more than she wanted to mention and felt she was an authority on diets. She also was not lacking in motivation. She claimed to have tried every diet out there and had been doing so for more than twenty years. Her weight: 250 pounds. That is a long time to be on a diet and not at your goal weight. No matter what the diet, Carol drank soda every day, thinking it wouldn't make a difference. I asked her how many she would have in a day, and she replied, "A couple of bottles."

Because one 16-ounce bottle of soda has about 200 calories, I found it hard to believe that two soft drinks would hinder her weight loss. My mistake was that I assumed she meant two 16-ounce bottles. She meant two 2-liter bottles per day! Clearly this was her diet vice and needed to be replaced with water.

Reluctantly, she took my advice and gave up her beloved soft drinks. After about six months, she called to tell me that she had been outside washing her car and started screaming. When her husband came running outside to rescue her, assuming that some kind of wild animal was attacking her, he found her jumping up and down and laughing. He asked what was wrong and she said that she was squatting down washing the tires when it hit her that she was squatting down! Something that, before busting her vice and losing 50 pounds, she hadn't done in years! Carol will be the first to tell you that she hadn't been dieting during that six months; what she had been doing was busting her soft drink vice and drinking a lot of water. What a difference one change can make.

Water will be decreasing the number of calories you consume each day because you will be replacing many, if not most, of the high-calorie drinks. Of course this is going to benefit you when you're trying to lose weight. You'll rid yourself of liquid calories, which are in the form of refined sugar—some of the worst. You will start to feel an immediate impact on your energy levels, and soon on your weight. You will be providing your body with a much-needed daily quantity of water.

As you move on into Week 2, continue to build this all-important habit. It can be the difference between a great deal of success and very little at all. And don't forget your affirmation.

 Daily Positive Affirmation

I have unlimited confidence in my abilities and myself. I am thankful for the endless opportunities that each day provides. I welcome optimal health into my life!

WEEK 2: BUSTING FAST FOOD
(AND OTHER FOOD VICES)

DAY 8

Actions: Continue to move toward the recommended intake of water each day.

For seven days you have focused on the one very important action of replacing unhealthy drinks with water. This week you'll be taking the first step in addressing the food in your diet—what you're eating that is the most responsible for your extra weight. You will need to put forth a bit more effort, engage in some planning, and exercise some willpower, but with this second step, you may just be putting yourself in a position to achieve more than 75 percent of your weight loss goals.

IDENTIFYING YOUR WORST FOOD VICE

For many people fast food is their diet vice. It's high in calories, consumed frequently and in quantity, isn't healthy, and is keeping them from losing weight. Now, fast food might not be your issue, or you may not have a *specific* food that you're eating too often or that has the most calories of all the foods you eat, but you can bet that you're eating *something* every day with little to no positive or healthy nutritional value that *is* negatively affecting your weight.

If it's not a specific food, then it may be one *food habit* that can be responsible for unneeded calories—like desserts after every lunch and dinner (even though it's a different one each day), or eating pastries for breakfast or a chocolate bar in the afternoon or snacking throughout the day.

The majority of people with whom I have worked, read about, or communicated with have a food that makes a difference in their weight. Surveys have shown that having a food vice is very real. So identifying what food or food habit you are indulging in regularly that is contributing the highest number of calories to your diet is important for taking steps toward losing weight.

Some of the most common food vices: cookies, muffins, desserts, pastries, potato chips, ice cream, chocolate, French fries, cereals, hot dogs, pasta, pizza, hamburgers, and cookie dough. The idea is to take a look at what your current diet consists of during a normal week and identify the food you consume on a fairly regular basis that is making a significant caloric contribution to your diet.

Take whatever time you need and identify your top food vice that contributes the most calories to your diet on a regular basis. Write that down here:

My food vice is: _____

This is the food (or habit) that you are going to **bust!**

✿ FOOD VICES

Some people feel that there is not one individual food that is a primary cause of their extra weight but rather a category or group of food like sweets, snacks, or breads.

What is common in all of these situations is the behavior you engage in regarding a certain food or a specific category of foods. It's something low in nutrition and high in calories that you eat regularly.

Eliminating Your Food Vice

Whether it's an individual food or a category of foods, this is contributing the most calories in your diet, and you must work on eliminating it or busting it. For those of you who might say you'd like to learn to eat a particular food in moderation, let me assure you that there are a few reasons it won't work. First, it is possible that the reason obesity statistics keeping getting higher is because we are kidding ourselves into believing that we can have our cake and eat it too. If we keep jumping from diet to diet, year after year, the real problem is that we just have not been told the truth about what it takes to reach a healthy weight. And the eating plans that we have been given with just about every diet are such a radical change from the foods we were (and still are) eating that there is just no way we can fathom giving them all up.

Another reason has to do with control. In order to have control over the (unhealthy) foods you eat, doesn't it make sense to first eliminate them to know if they are or are not controlling you? (After you complete this plan, if you find that you want to reintroduce particular foods into your diet, you are welcome to try but it is my advice not to do so. You are better off without a particular food that you can't handle in "moderation" than constantly trying to have it in "moderation" and failing. I eliminated ice cream from my life a decade ago and I have not consumed any since. I decided that I did not want to eat something that really has no value to my health and contributed to my being overweight. If you're serious about losing weight, then do what it takes to get there.) I have found that most people can handle this approach so much better than any other approach they've tried. I believe the same will hold true for you. Simple works: eliminate one food item and replace it with a healthy substitute.

Substituting Healthy Beverages and Foods

When you eliminate your **food vice**, it's time to find something healthy that you are going to eat in place of it. Following is a list of healthy substitutes that you can choose from, or you can come up with your own. This will obviously be a food item to help your weight loss efforts but that also will support a healthy lifestyle.

1. Acceptable Healthy Beverages

water—90% of total beverage intake
green tea, unsweetened
milk, skim or 1%
orange, apple, grape juice (not from concentrate)—8 ounces per
    day
coffee—if you must have, use no sweeteners or sugar substitutes

2. Some Recommended *Diet Vice* Replacement Foods*

apples†	raisins	turkey breast
oranges†	popcorn (no salt, no	12-grain bread
grapes†	butter)	natural unsweetened
bananas†	brown rice†	applesauce
baby carrots†	salads†	Egg Beaters
pineapple	lean meats	butter substitutes
grapefruit	white fish	Yoplait Lite yogurt
carrots	rice cakes	bean soup
celery	artichokes	
tomatoes	deli sandwiches with	
pears	lean meat	
plums	grilled chicken breast	

3. Other suggestions

cold cereals: Kashi Go-Lean—add milled flaxseeds and wheat
   germ
low-sugar Gum
honey
protein shakes—I like Juice Plus+ Complete®—Vanilla

When you remove something from your life, especially a habit, you need to fill that space or time with something else. You will do that instinctively, whether you think you have to or not. (This is many times true for those who overeat after a divorce—they find they're filling the time or a void in their life by eating instead.) Because your body needs some nutrition—especially if you're going to replace an unhealthy meal—you need to find a healthy substitute. There are a few different variables here related to what, when, and how much you're eating that we need to concern ourselves with, but let's start with the basic principle.

First, you need to estimate the amount of healthy food you need to substitute. If you have been consuming an entire meal—fast food, for

---

*These are healthier substitutes, but do not eat unlimited quantities. There are many other healthier food choices that qualify—just be sure the quantity is reasonable.
†Julia's favorites

example—then you have to devise some healthy substitutes to replace it. Of course, you probably don't want to make some extreme changes regarding the quantity of food you're used to consuming or the time you're going to eat, or how long it takes to make your meal, especially when you've been accustomed to getting it fast. You don't need to calculate and weigh the exact number of calories and size, which most diets require. You can adjust the course of your life just a degree or two, so that every time you would normally indulge in **unhealthy** fast food, you will now get a **healthier version** of fast food.

In other words, consider the options that are available. If you have to grab a meal on the run, go to a deli where you can get a fresh and healthier sandwich. Or try precooked meals from the supermarket that include chicken, fish, rice, or lean beef and vegetables. Remember, you are changing one meal each day, not the entire day's meals. Remember, it's not necessary to count the number of calories you were consuming and what this new meal contains. Consume about the same portion size for now, and choose something other than the hamburger, hot dog, or other fat-laden foods that you were eating. Find places in your community where you can get a healthy meal *fast* so that the habit only changes from bad to good, as opposed to a completely different routine (for now anyway). Subway, for example, is a much better option than the typical fast-food establishment.

Another option, of course, is to have a healthier meal planned in place of your usual stop or drive-through. If you can plan in advance for the coming week, you'll be much better off, whether it's food you prepare in advance or something you pick up. (See the recipe section, Appendix II, page 179, for some ideas.)

If you are eating a particular food item or too much of a certain category of items, you may find making substitutions a little bit easier. If you can identify one food that needs to be busted, you don't have to worry (yet) about replacing an entire meal. Either way, you need to **work on eliminating that item and replacing it with a healthy substitute**. Because most people don't get enough fruits or vegetables in their diet, I recommend choosing one or two that you know you enjoy and make it the item that you'll eat in place of your busted food. There are plenty of fruits to choose from, and some vegetables, that have a variety of tastes and also will appeal to your palate.

Have a Healthy Snack

The smartest, most logical, and tasty suggestion that I can make as you bust your food vice is to find two or three fruits and a couple of vegetables that taste good to you and get in the habit of keeping some of them on hand during the day. I found that I could snack on baby carrots instead of my usual bag of candy. This not only reduced my appetite and made me feel a whole lot better, but I also wasn't sluggish toward the end of the afternoon. In fact, carrots have plenty of necessary fiber and vitamins. In retrospect, I think I was providing my body with a much-needed cleansing with all of the fiber I was getting. You can do the same thing with any fruit or vegetable. Use it as a food to snack on during the day, which not only replaces your food vice but will help reduce your appetite come mealtime. This is the easiest, most effective way to cut out your food vice while providing yourself with a needed fruit or vegetable.

The most important way to think about this step is to try to keep it simple. You can't ignore the fact that you're already doing things a certain way and probably have been for a long time. So you can effectively make these changes **only if** you can do them gradually—one change at a time over a longer period, as opposed to a massive lifestyle overhaul in the first day. Focus on replacing one unhealthy food or food item (high in fat or total calories) that you are consuming too much of on a regular basis. Choose one or two healthy substitutes to eat in place of these unhealthy items. Try to make that one change and work on doing it each day.

 Daily Positive Affirmation
I have unlimited confidence in my abilities and myself. I am thankful for the endless opportunities that each day provides. I welcome optimal health into my life!

Day 9

Actions: (1) Continue to move toward the recommended intake of water each day; (2) Substitute healthy food(s) in place of your *food vice.*

One of the first issues raised when it comes to eliminating the unhealthy fast food or the cookies, chocolates, or ice cream is whether it is necessary to completely remove the food from the diet. Many people have turned down this approach because they don't think they need to completely give up the foods they like. While I'm not saying you can't enjoy food, the problem is that you may have been enjoying it too much at the expense of healthy eating. You need to eat to fuel your body and its functions, and while eating is pleasurable, I can't tell you that it's okay to have some of this or a little bit of that. If you have some, you'll probably want more! It is very, very difficult to have just one bite of the food you love without slipping back to old habits you formed from foods and beverages that are **addictive**.

At first you may think you are being deprived mentally and physically, but by giving up one food item, there is a lot to be gained. Have you been depriving yourself of a healthy and fit lifestyle because of extra calories? Is this a food that has been providing you with the pain, the sadness, and the frustration of carrying weight you don't want or need? Have you been losing time, energy, productivity, and money at your job because of this diet vice? Do you want to spend more time with your spouse traveling, going out, or even having more sexual relations than you do now but aren't because of this diet vice (even indirectly)? I think it's safe to say that there are no positive benefits to keeping your food vice around anymore; don't you agree?

Deprivation is not living without an unhealthy food. It's living with it and not being able to enjoy life at a healthy weight, with a more fit body that is more energetic. Deprivation is keeping yourself from doing so many things that you should be able to do—that *you want to do*—but don't because of the extra weight. The only time deprivation exists is when you continue to choose unhealthy over healthy. That will deprive you of your true potential. If you live with a known preventable barrier between who you are now and who you would like to be, it is your responsibility to do something about it.

Lose the unhealthy food permanently and replace it with a healthy food. You will be choosing a life of fulfillment and happiness. Leave the unhealthy behind and make it symbolic of leaving behind any disappointments, frustrations, or anger that you've had in the past. Welcome the energy, fulfillment, and new potential that lie ahead.

Valerie is a woman in her twenties who had been living with a few bad habits—one of which was cupcakes each day. After having identified this vice and realizing that she needed to start with one change, she went on to lose 150-plus pounds over the next few months. It was breaking her sweet tooth that gave her the needed start in the right direction and eventually led to her to lose the weight. Living with those habits was keeping her from so many things—and she's now living her dreams! It just takes a step in the right direction, and if you continue with this second step you will see more and more positive benefits.

 Daily Positive Affirmation
I have unlimited confidence in my abilities and myself. I am thankful for the endless opportunities that each day provides. I welcome optimal health into my life!

DAY 10

Actions: (1) Carry a water bottle with you and drink plenty of water; (2) Substitute a healthy food in place of your *food vice*.

If you were on a boat in the middle of the ocean and you were traveling 10 miles per hour and changed your course by 1 degree, the next week you would be miles away from where you were headed had you not changed your course. A small change can, over time, make a big change. To succeed on this plan only a few changes are really necessary to get to a healthy weight (or at least close).

AN eDIETS.COM SURVEY

The Web site eDiets.com, the home to more than fourteen million subscribers who are seeking better health and fitness, did a survey to find out more about their subscribers' diet vices. They asked the readers, "Do you have diet vices?" and "If so, what are they?" Also, "How many times a day or week do you break your diet to indulge in them?" And finally, "Do you feel guilty about cheating on your diet?"

The responses were quite interesting.

- 91 percent of the respondents said yes, they had diet vices.
- The most common answers given were: candy or chocolate, fast food, pizza, potato chips, cookies, ice cream, and soft drinks.
- 38 percent said that they stray off their plan DAILY while another 33 percent claim to do so WEEKLY. That makes 71 percent of dieters whose vices are controlling their lives and hindering their weight loss efforts.
- 81 percent of the respondents felt guilty about giving in to their vices.

Reading these statistics convinced me of two things: we are not alone in our struggles with these vice foods, and vice busting is essential if we are ever to lose weight and keep it off.

It does you no good to go on a diet that prescribes a recommended eating plan if you are just going to go off it to indulge in your vices. It makes much more sense to rid your life of the vices that continually sabotage your efforts. The food that contributes the most calories to your diet on the most frequent basis is your vice.

The USDA has reported that a large percentage of the increase in calories in our diets from 1978 to 1996 comes from the increased consumption of snacks. You wouldn't expect a recovering alcoholic to take a job in a bar serving alcohol, so you shouldn't expect to go to a restaurant, where 90 percent of the foods are fattening, unhealthy, and quite possibly addictive. The only sure way to avoid those extra calories is to stay away.

This is why it is important to work on just that one food or those daily snacks that come from the quick-stop shops. You don't need them; they aren't doing anything but satisfying a desire. Break it, tear it, crush it, stomp it, throw it, burn it. **BUST IT!** You can do it!

 Daily Positive Affirmation

I have unlimited confidence in my abilities and myself. I am thankful for the endless opportunities that each day provides. I welcome optimal health into my life!

DAY 11

Actions: (1) Carry a water bottle with you and drink plenty of water; (2) Substitute a healthy food in place of your *food vice*.

Do a self-evaluation as you move on each day. Hold yourself accountable for your own success. If you know you missed this morning's usual intake of water because you forgot your water bottle, be aware of that fact but don't beat yourself up about it. However, if you continued without water or ate your food vice, maybe you're not putting in an honest effort. Building your awareness is an important part of the process. I used a 32-ounce bottle of water and emptied it at least twice a day. Drinking water is such a habit now that I can tell if I'm not getting enough water by the way I feel. As far as vice food goes, it's important to be prepared to avoid "the enemy." The best defense is a strong offense. If you're prepared, your temptation and your previous bad habit have a fraction of a chance to survive.

We all need to regularly look at what we're doing that is good. You may not see the changes in your body, but being focused on the two simple actions that you should be doing at this point is what's important. Each day if you take the time to reflect on the good decisions you're making, you can reinforce the positive steps you're taking.

- Do I feel that my actions to eliminate unhealthy foods are a responsible decision?
- Am I going through the motions because that's what the plan says to do?
- Am I motivated to change for the better and improve more than just my weight?
- Do I believe that a few simple changes can really improve my life?
- Do I care enough about my future to put forth a positive and honest effort?
- Will I realize more satisfaction and fulfillment by living healthy all the time?
- Why did I eat my food vice or drink a soda?

These types of questions will help you decide whether you are motivated to be in this for the long haul. That is not to say that you won't have any slip-ups or setbacks, because we all do. When you start to think about your overall future and the consequences of remaining where you are now versus where you *can be,* then you will stay motivated.

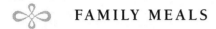 **FAMILY MEALS**

Most often we are feeding the kids (and our spouses) what we are eating, or vice versa: we're eating what our spouses feed us. Many people will explain to me that they can't give up a certain thing because it is always in the house. Well, aren't your kids and spouse entitled to a healthy diet? With what you now know you can help your family eat and live healthily.

I hope you have let them know that water is good for them and that they should be increasing the amount they drink while decreasing their consumption of unhealthy beverages. Obesity doesn't discriminate, and today more children than ever before are obese. Adult-onset diabetes is now referred to as type 2 diabetes because children and teenagers are getting it at an epidemic rate. We are starting to see hypertension and cardiac problems in younger and younger people as well. Make your family part of the reason you need to get healthy so you can continue making the necessary changes.

Peggy talked with me after seven days of *vice-busting.* She said it was a little bit difficult at first, but she managed to stick with it and get over the hump. She said she felt that she should be doing much more because she was on a diet. I assured her she didn't need to do more now but would eventually. I asked her why she felt that way, because it wasn't clear to me if she just wanted to see more results (we're talking about only one week here!). It was actually just the opposite—she felt so good that she wanted to do more. That was a relief. Although I was happy to hear about her success, I told her it was important to continue to do what was planned so that these actions would become habits, not just a temporary move to lose weight (which would then also be temporary). After many months, she is happy to be living at a healthy weight, without doing anything strenuous or complicated.

Daily Positive Affirmation
I have unlimited confidence in my abilities and myself. I am
thankful for the endless opportunities that each day provides.
I welcome optimal health into my life!

DAY 12

Actions: (1) Carry a water bottle with you and drink plenty of water;
(2) Substitute a healthy food in place of your *food vice*.

A bottle of water each day, and a piece of fruit or a packed lunch
in place of your food vice, are what these first two weeks are about.
Each day is a chance to do one thing that, over time, will make a difference.

Not too long ago, one of my family members mentioned to me that
he needed to reduce his cholesterol level. The doctor told him that his
triglyceride levels were ten times higher than what is suggested, and his
cholesterol was elevated about 20 percent above the upper limits.
While diet and genetics play a part in cholesterol issues, I was curious
about his situation, because he was not obviously overweight. He was
embarking on a diet plan reluctantly because he didn't want to start
eating different foods, many of which he didn't like or know how to
prepare. Rather than go on an extreme diet, I told him to look at *the
changes* that his doctor suggested he make and break them down to one
change a week. Also, that he needed to think of them as a lifestyle
change. Now he has a healthier level of both triglycerides and cholesterol, and his eating habits (diet) are enjoyable and *healthy*.

 ## IMPROVE YOUR HEALTH WITH
FRUITS AND VEGETABLES

It is possible to be at or near a healthy weight and have cholesterol problems, which tells me that our diet is hurting more of us
than those who are overweight.

If you add up the calories from each food group that you eat in one day, I'm willing to bet that the lowest percentage of those comes from fruit or vegetables and the highest comes from breads, fats, and meats. It is much easier to get many calories from a small amount of fat but it would take a lot of carrots, celery, broccoli, or tomatoes to get the same amount. Even fruits like apples, oranges, strawberries, and grapes would require a large amount to equal the calories in a small portion of a fatty food. Another benefit from eating the proper amount of fruits and vegetables is the fiber that it adds to your diet.

Some plans advocate avoiding sugar entirely, but not all sugars are the same. If you eat the natural source of sugar that comes directly from an apple or an orange, for example, then you aren't going to be hurting your health. On the contrary, it will be helpful. Start picking up more fruits and using them as your snack food, or your replacement for your food vice. Remember, our survey from eDiets.com revealed some of the most common food vices to be chips, candy, and cookies. All of these foods can be replaced with a piece of fruit, or even a vegetable. Don't wait to make a big change; take one more healthy action than you were doing two weeks ago.

 ## COUNT YOUR BLESSINGS

One of the most important exercises you can do to improve your outlook while building and maintaining a positive mental attitude (PMA) is to take note of the things you have to be thankful for. It can be difficult when you're overweight to overcome mental hurdles or blocks that get in the way of weight loss. But a change of mind can make big changes in life. In fact, 98 percent of life's challenges consist primarily of **mental challenges.** When you are faced with having to accomplish a task or goal, the overwhelming percentage of your efforts usually has to do with making a plan of attack and having the conviction that you can be successful. The rest is just doing.

One way you can start to believe in yourself is to look around to see what it is, in fact, that makes you happy. What people, places, things, events, jobs, sights, pictures, memories, and anything else that is close to your heart can you appreciate in some way? You may some-times forget about all of the great things in your life because you become so focused on your looks and your weight. Make today a day to appreciate the bounty in your life.

What experiences have you had in the last year, or five or ten, that you have enjoyed? It can be as simple as a child or grandchild's sporting event or as exciting as a tour of Europe. If you're having trouble counting your blessings, following are some ideas to get you thinking.

I Can Be Thankful For:

children	holidays	nourishment	literacy
my spouse	having choices	opportunities	knowledge
laughter	snow days	creative ideas	my best friend
light	ice skating	airplanes	my religion
a warm home	salads	movies	technology
my car	my cell phone	fruits	my computer
my job	playgrounds	cartoons	a scented
friendships	my relatives'	water filters	candle
love/marriage	kids	fresh sheets	a friendly smile
sunlight	birthdays	a warm towel	a stranger's help
beaches	(mine, too!)	good music	volunteers
vacations	a hot bath	a sparkling fire	the gift of life
family	clothing/outfits	the zoo	

 Daily Positive Affirmation
I have unlimited confidence in my abilities and myself. I am thankful for the endless opportunities that each day provides. I welcome optimal health into my life!

Day 13

Actions: (1) Carry a water bottle with you and drink plenty of water; (2) Substitute a healthy food in place of your *food vice.*

I hope you feel as though you have made some good changes in your life. I also hope you have noticed the absence of an eating plan, and also the lack of emphasis on food. If you are constantly focused on everything you need to eat, and everything you shouldn't eat, then you will remain focused on the problem—food. The solution is to focus on some simple actions to get started, and on the short-term goals (completing your actions for the day and for the week).

THREE REASONS FOR OBESITY

I believe that we, as a country, our failing to reach a healthy weight for three reasons.

First, we routinely eat what we like and like what we eat. Because so many people are doing it, it can't be that bad, can it? I wonder if you are among the people included in the statistics of high cholesterol, high blood pressure, or the gamut of health concerns more likely to result from being overweight. I've heard that millions of people may be walking around who have no idea that they are diabetic. By taking the steps during this week to break a food vice, you should be learning a lot about yourself. Each day you may be tempted by whatever it is, but believe me, it's not worth it. Keep your focus on where you *want* and *need* to go.

The **second** reason we may be missing the boat when it comes to our health is that we are simply misinformed about the dangers of eating a large majority of the foods available to us. Just about every restaurant has a menu on which unhealthy items outweigh the healthy. Most items have too much bread, butter, salt, creamy sauce, batter, grease, oil, fat, or are served in too large a portion. If you want to indulge there are much better things to indulge in.

The **third** reason the obesity statistics continue to rise is because of our lack of goals—yearly, monthly, weekly, and even daily goals. I believe that we are just bored. We don't have things to do that we could and should be doing, because we don't have a list of what it is we'd like to get done. Are there things around your house that *you'd* like to get done? Are there some things you've forgotten about? What about something that you've been wanting to do with your kids? Do you have an interest in something that you have put off? Ask yourself why you've put it off. Do you have any excuses that are just so you don't have to take action now? Set a goal and take action!

BREAK THE CYCLE, EDUCATE YOURSELF, SET GOALS

To overcome the forces that conspire to keep you fat you need to counter them. The first step is to break the cycle (the habit). In order to break the cycle, you're going to change your course a bit.

The second thing you need to do is to educate yourself about what's healthy and what's not.

The third thing you need to do is to set goals. Solidify in your mind *what it is that you* really *want*. Remember, it's not only a better body that you seek, but the things you think will happen for you as a result of only having a better body. It's not necessarily having more energy that you want, it's the things that you believe you will be able to do with more energy that you aren't doing now. Setting clear goals will give you a clearer vision of where you are going.

 Daily Positive Affirmation

I have unlimited confidence in my abilities and myself. I am thankful for the endless opportunities that each day provides. I welcome optimal health into my life!

DAY 14

Actions: (1) Carry a water bottle with you and drink plenty of water; (2) Substitute a healthy food in place of your *food vice*.

At the end of two weeks the changes that you will feel at this point—mentally, emotionally, physically, and possibly spiritually—should be noticeable. If not, let's just say that you have not moved as quickly as you would have liked. The good news is that this isn't a race. You can set the pace that's most comfortable and effective for you.

✢ WEEK 2 REVIEW

Today's self-evaluation will help to determine the strengths of your actions and of the areas that need improving.

How do I feel about my progress up to this point?
How does my body feel now compared to when I started?
Can I do more to improve upon what I have done so far?
Is this something I think I can do for the rest of my life?
Do I feel deprived or empowered?

These questions are strictly meant for the purpose of strengthening your mental resolve to improve your life. If you can give a positive answer to at least three of the five then you have made progress.

✢ FOOD IS FUEL

Do we ever stop to think that the food we need is merely fuel to keep our body functioning healthily? In many ways, it's no different from purchasing high quality gasoline to run our automobiles. Our taste buds have become a *pleasure gauge* rather than a *quality gauge*. We no longer look for the taste that is healthy (void of too much salt, sugar, or spice), but instead become more focused on how pleasing the food is to our palate. Food and drinks have become things of pleasure and are no longer viewed just as a source of needed fuel.

It is *satisfying* to have a good meal when you're hungry and you've worked hard all day. It is not a reward, but a time to reflect on a busy and productive day while getting your necessary nutrition. However, choosing unhealthy foods and snacks to eat throughout the day that are not necessary (because you're not hungry and/or don't need those types of foods) is taking that *satisfaction* to a point of *indulging* in pleasure. There is nothing wrong with enjoying the time taken to sit down, relax, socialize, and eat a meal. But if you keep your perspective on what you **need** for your body, you'll **want** less and less of those things that are unhealthy and not needed.

WHERE YOU ARE NOW

First, water should be a part of your life throughout the day every day. You should be carrying a water bottle with you and having it within reach almost all of the time.

Start your morning by drinking an 8-ounce glass of water. One glass will be out of the way before you even begin your day. You are going to be amazed at how you will soon, if you don't already, crave water.

"The secret to shedding pounds may be in a glass of water. Drink the right amount of water and you'll burn more calories." That is what scientists at Berlin's Franz-Volhard Clinic Research Center have to say about water. They have scientifically shown that people who drink two liters of water a day burn an extra 150 calories daily. Their findings show that water apparently seems to stimulate the sympathetic nerve system that regulates metabolism, and that people who drink 500 milligrams of water increase their metabolic rate by 30 percent. Your metabolic rate is the rate at which calories are burned. Interestingly, as much as 40 percent of the increase in calorie burning is caused by your body's attempt to heat the water you just drank!

Also, they say that you should drink good old-fashioned water: carbonated water and all the other flavored waters, including soft drinks, actually have a negative effect on metabolic rates (as reported in the *Journal of Clinical Endocrinology & Metabolism*). So continue working on building the habit of making water your beverage of choice 90 percent or more of the time.

Secondly, you should realize by now whether your food vice has had control over your weight in the past. At the one-week point I notice many people begin to have a difficult time giving up their food vice. There is a point where your mind may tell you it's okay to have "just a bite" or "just one." These urges may be tough to ward off, but you've got to do it. The only way you know that you are in control is to say no, at least for now. Whether it be fast food, a specific item (like cookies), a category of items (all sweets, for example), or just portion sizes (eating too much, too often), you've got to stick to your resolve to eliminate the bad and replace it with the good. As a reminder, here are some examples of common **food vices** and their healthy replacements.

Vice-Food Eliminated	Healthy Replacement
fast food	healthy salad/small deli sandwich
pizza	low-fat oat muffin
cookies	baby carrots
chocolate	apples or oranges
candy bars	celery with low-fat peanut butter
potato chips	grapes or apples
high-sugar cereal	oatmeal or egg whites
fast-food breakfast	all-fiber cereal with wheat germ
desserts, pies	bowl of assorted fruit
pastries	fruits
hamburgers	grilled chicken

 Daily Positive Affirmation

I have unlimited confidence in my abilities and myself. I am thankful for the endless opportunities that each day provides. I welcome optimal health into my life!

WEEK 3: BUSTING TELEVISION

DAY 15

Actions: (1) Carry a water bottle with you and drink plenty of water; (2) Substitute a healthy food in place of your *food vice.*

It may seem odd to focus on television in a weight loss plan but it fits the definition of **a habitual action that keeps you from reaching and maintaining a healthy weight.** The hours you spend in front of the television are keeping you from doing productive things, like using your imagination to come up with new ideas, inventions, approaches, techniques, solutions to your own problems or situations—or even to those problems that exist on a global scale.

It's possible that television is just as addictive as some of the foods available to us. How else could it be that we are watching (using?) it four hours a day? There are plenty of other exciting, fascinating, exhil-arating, and productive things that we can do. I'm not suggesting that you eliminate TV entirely, but that you use it more judiciously and per-haps at the same time as you engage in some calorie-burning exercise.

 ADDING EXERCISE FOR LIFE

In order to improve your health and fitness, it is necessary to incorporate *exercise* into your life, and because the action this week is about TV, you must begin to enforce a new rule as you make the transi-tion to a healthy and fit lifestyle: **No TV unless you've already done, or are doing, some exercise.**

That does not that mean that you have to exercise at all times you normally watch TV. It means that if you are going to watch television then you need to have completed your exercise for the day.

Exercise has got to be a part of your daily life in order for you to be healthy and fit.

One of the easiest ways to get started exercising (or to increase the time you now exercise) is to do it while watching TV. If you have one TV show you enjoy, why not plan to be doing something while you're watching? If it's possible, go to your gym and walk, jog, or run (depending on your health and fitness level) on the treadmill while your favorite show airs. Not only will you not have to give up watching TV, but you can focus on something entertaining while you exercise.

An Easy Approach to Exercise

Whether you are currently exercising or following an exercise program, it is important that you read through this section and absorb the content. Many people shy away from, or just plain hate to, exercise, because it seems too difficult. The solution is finding the right type of exercise for you and making it enjoyable.

If you've tried to do some form of exercise and stopped, you may have found that it was too complicated or painful. However, the problem was not with you but with the approach. Too often we get started on a new exercise program, machine, or technique, only to burn out after a few days because we've overdone it, or tried to do too much too soon. You can't develop the habit of exercising on a regular basis if you don't start on a level that's comfortable for you.

It is important to know your health and fitness level so that you can determine what exercises you should be starting with and to have a vision of what it is going to take to get to your desired level of fitness. Appendix I further explain levels of fitness. For now, suffice it to say that your goal should be to move at least three times a week. You can walk, take a class at the Y or gym, or work out at home to an exercise video you love. Of course, you should check in with your doctor before engaging in any exercise program.

Overcoming the "Stopping Factors"

Listening to music is also a great way to keep you focused on moving forward. The beat of the music will help you keep pace and keep moving as long as the music keeps playing. Music can also block out what I call "stopping factors" or the things that make you want to stop exercising.

After exercising for a few minutes, as your heart starts beating faster, your breathing increases, and you begin perspiring, your mind can begin to wander. You may start to think about everything other than where you are and what you are doing. As you continue, you may feel your heart beating a little harder and faster, you may hear yourself breathing faster and a little louder, and you may feel the perspiration and your body heating up. Your mind may wander a bit more. This can create stopping factors. These may be fear, thinking you are too much out of shape and could get hurt; or anxiety, because the physical changes are unfamiliar to you; or even insecurity, because you don't see yourself as a "fitness person." The negative chatter may rev up, telling you that you need to be doing something else or be somewhere else, taking your mind off exercise and consuming your thoughts. These are just normal psychological influences that occur because you're putting your body under stress (although it is good stress), and giving your brain freshly oxygenated blood, which will get you thinking even more!

Caution: if you feel faint or out of breath, slow down and cool down so you can regain your breath. Do not push yourself beyond your limits.

Some people stop exercising just as they are getting started as a defense mechanism to avoid being "overworked." If you stop, you may just quit before you've given yourself the chance to reach that fat-burning level and that feel-good level. By listening to music with headphones or ear pieces you can drown out the sounds of being tired and other distractions, all the while focusing on the sounds of your music (or TV). If you can use ear pieces to listen to the TV or music while you're exercising, you'll find a big difference in your ability to go the duration without stopping for twenty, thirty, forty-five minutes or more. Put all your favorite songs on a disk or download to your iPod for ease.

Remember, this isn't about overdoing it; it's just about getting around the psychological blocks that you very often put up because many of these exercises you just may not like doing (at first)!

❧ OUTLOOK FOR WEEK 3

It is important that you have at least three days of exercise scheduled this week. First, be sure to determine what kind of exercise is most suitable for you based on your health and fitness levels (see Appendix I, page 165). Next, decide when you're going to do it, then how many days this week are most appropriate. Plan on how much time you'll need to exercise. The key here is to start with a reasonable schedule as well as a reasonable workout plan. As time goes on, you can incorporate greater duration, more intensity, and higher frequency to your exercise.

If you are already going to the gym and are trying to lose those last 20 pounds, you may already be ahead of the game. But it is important that you follow along with this entire plan because it is not a short-term change; you will be incorporating good habits into your routine so that you won't ever again have to worry about an extra 20 pounds.

Keep affirming the positive.

 Daily Positive Affirmation

I have unlimited confidence in my abilities and myself. I am thankful for the endless opportunities that each day provides. I welcome optimal health into my life!

DAY 16

Actions: (1) Carry a water bottle with you and drink plenty of water; (2) Substitute a healthy food in place of your *food vice*; (3) Replace sedentary TV time with exercise.

You have eliminated soft drinks or other high-sugar, high-calorie drinks and replaced them with water; you have eliminated your worst and highest-calorie food (or meal) and replaced it with a healthy one; and you have started to incorporate exercise into your life. These are three important actions that can make all the difference in the world when measuring your health and fitness level. These three habits can and will create a ripple effect into other areas of your diet and your life as you will see in the coming weeks. This week, you should focus on making time to exercise on a regular basis.

MAKE EXERCISE A HABIT

If you have never before taken the time to do any form of exercise—or have done so sporadically in the past—the most important step you can take *right now* is to set your schedule. Make your appointment for physical activity so you know you have an hour set aside at least three times this week. You will have a routine of taking an hour to focus on nothing but exercise. Make it a new good habit.

Once you have your schedule set, stick with it. Write it in your calendar, make it part of your day. Soon it will become automatic.

FIND A PARTNER . . .

There are many benefits of having someone with you while working out, whether it's a friend or someone in an exercise class. Having someone with you to walk, talk, and focus on reaching the end point makes working out a whole lot easier. Also, if you've arranged to meet someone for a walk or a class you'll be less likely to not show up, because you'll be disappointing a friend, as well as letting yourself down.

An exercise partner . . .

keeps you accountable
provides you with company
helps get you motivated
brings on competition
inspires you to succeed
contributes new ideas
supports a healthy diet
desires a common goal(s)
celebrates your success

And, of course, **you** do the same for them!

With one or more other people working, exercising, or striving to reach the same goal, the effort becomes easier even though the work is the same. If you aren't at the level of health and fitness now that brings you to the gym for group exercise classes, start to think about and visualize becoming part of a regular schedule so that you will see some of the same people being your support (and you theirs), all in the name of good health.

 TRANSITION TO FITNESS

While you are beginning to implement this third and important habit into your lifestyle, keep in mind the *suitable transition* that is necessary to establish the habit. Review the three components to making exercise an integral part of your life:

1. Choose exercises from *your* level of health and fitness.
2. Schedule a time you will commit to regularly.
3. Gradually increase frequency, duration, and intensity.

 Daily Positive Affirmation

I have unlimited confidence in my abilities and myself. I am thankful for the endless opportunities that each day provides. I welcome optimal health into my life!

DAY 17

Actions: (1) Carry a water bottle with you and drink plenty of water; (2) Substitute a healthy food in place of your *food vice*; (3) Replace sedentary TV time with exercise.

You should be feeling the physical and mental changes that accompany the first two actions. You may be just starting to exercise this week for the first time or for the first time in what seems like a long time. Either way all you should do now is focus on going forward because there is no going back. Where you may have failed before, you shouldn't be straining to succeed now. Continue to focus on the actions that you need to do today and today only, while you visualize a life full of fitness, free from sickness, and filled with vigor.

This week is devoted to busting the television habit in favor of exercise. Reducing your TV watching can also keep you from being exposed to bad news, which will inevitably bring you down.

By Replacing TV with Exercise You Will

1. limit the bad news let into your mind;
2. provide freshly oxygenated blood to your brain;
3. release endorphins and enkephalins* into your body.

When you perform sustained physical activity for at least thirty minutes, your heart will pump a little faster and a bit harder, and your breathing will increase in rate and volume. This is your body's way of getting the oxygen (among other things) to the muscles, organs, and tissues that will sustain your exertion. Eventually, endorphins and enkephalins (one sooner, one later) are released into your body's bloodstream, which will make you feel good due to their *analgesic properties*.

 ## NEW GUIDELINES

In 2005, the United States Department of Agriculture (USDA) released its new guidelines for eating and maintaining health. Without going into all of the details, the biggest standout among the changes is the recommendation for more exercise. The USDA suggests spending thirty minutes each day on physical activity and sixty to ninety minutes if you want to lose weight.

The overall guideline for exercise has changed because we have become so sedentary over the past twenty years. The only way to make up for more time sitting is to spend more time devoted to sustained exercising.

---

*Neurotransmitters that are released in your body and inhibit the pain signal to the brain.

On the vice-busting plan, the goal is to eventually have thirty minutes per day for at least five days a week, each week. When you exercise according to this plan for a sustained amount of time you can almost be guaranteed to improve your health. Although exercise provides many healthy benefits, keep in mind that they don't happen overnight.

No matter what level of health and fitness that you are on, if you don't feel like exercising, get up and take a walk for ten minutes. You can always increase your time and/or distance as you get used to incorporating exercise into your routine.

USING A PEDOMETER

An easy and convenient tool to help you monitor physical activity is a digital pedometer that will measure the number of steps you take each day. It attaches to your waistband or belt buckle and is very lightweight.

Wearing a pedometer is like having your own personal trainer providing immediate feedback on your activity level. It's a great way to find out if you're getting the recommended number of steps and/or thirty minutes of daily activity recommended by the U.S. surgeon general. Studies show that a pedometer raises both your awareness and the actual amount of your daily activity. Wear it for a few days to establish your baseline—to see how many steps you take during one of your "normal" days. Then make an effort to increase your steps by 10 percent per week.

A pedometer really is the best tool to heighten your awareness, and I consider it an essential, must-have item.

 Daily Positive Affirmation

I have unlimited confidence in my abilities and myself. I am thankful for the endless opportunities that each day provides. I welcome optimal health into my life!

Day 18

Actions: (1) Carry a water bottle with you and drink plenty of water; (2) Substitute a healthy food in place of your *food vice;* (3) Replace sedentary TV time with exercise.

One common lapse that I have noted with many people at this point is a slip in their conviction to completely eliminate their diet vices. They believe, "If I have just one, it'll be okay and won't get me off track." Let me tell you right now, one *will* get you off track. The problem with this type of thinking (at least at this point) is that you haven't yet learned to do without the food(s) and drink(s) that you really have no business consuming anyway.

❧ A NEED OR A WANT

Anytime you think you can reach for one _____ (fill in the blank) then think to yourself, "Is this something I want or something I *need*?" You'll discover that you just *want* it instead of *need* it. This is the **tough love** part of this plan—you've got to stick to your resolve to completely rid yourself of what is unhealthy in order to reach optimal health. And the steps to this plan are only the basic ones to get you started in that direction. Again, each day as you continue with this plan, ask yourself:

1. **Is this a *need* or is this a *want*?**
2. **Will this increase/decrease my level of health?**

You can save yourself a lot of pain if you refer to these questions when you're making choices. Eventually **you will want those things that you need!** And that is the lifestyle you are striving to achieve. Your mind, body, and spirit will be more balanced and motivated to seek out what's healthy all the time.

Let's review three important reasons that it's necessary to follow the **No TV until exercise** rule:

1. *If you think you can do what you've always done and get a different result you are going to be let down.* If you travel the same route every day and always hit the same big pothole that gives you a flat tire, then you'll probably find the same sad result if you don't alter your path.

2. *If you get comfortable watching your favorite show, it can turn into watching TV for the next two hours.* By sticking to the **No TV until exercise** rule, you'll avoid this trap.

3. *It puts your priorities in order of importance.* You must put exercise, and your health, ahead of TV on the scale of importance. If you want to reach other goals—social, financial, spiritual, personal, political, whatever—and think that exercise should be second, then you may just be losing **a lot** for other, undesirable gains.

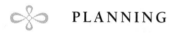 ## PLANNING

Planning what to eat ahead of time will be instrumental in keeping you away from unhealthy choices. There are three things to plan for at this point: (1) be sure you have enough water with you at all times; (2) have your healthy food(s) purchased and part of your diet whether it is for your snack, for a meal, or taken with you to work; (3) you should know what exercise you will be doing and when and where you will be doing it. Having a plan in place will be a tremendous help toward reaching your goal—and staying there!

To track your progress and keep your plan in place, use a daily planner and write down what you need to do each day and for the week. In addition to your steps toward weight loss, fill in the blanks with every other chore, task, or project that you need to focus on—for work, home, family, and so on.

Using a daily planner will help you know what you're doing with your time and whether you actually have more time during the day than you thought. I often hear people tell me that they don't have time to go to the gym. My usually comeback is, "You don't have time not to." There is not enough time to waste on unhealthy living and unhealthy choices. Take the guesswork out of having to find the time. Write down what you *have to* get done today, what you *need to* get done today, and what you *want to* get done today—and when you plan on doing each. You'll then know what your commitment level is for all of the things on your list. Then at the end of a month, you don't have to get on the scale to know your progress; you can just look at whether you completed the healthy things you had planned each day for the past month. In this way, you will be holding *yourself* accountable for doing the steps in this plan *and* those in every other area of your life.

 Daily Positive Affirmation
I have unlimited confidence in my abilities and myself. I am thankful for the endless opportunities that each day provides. I welcome optimal health into my life!

Day 19

Actions: (1) Carry a water bottle with you and drink plenty of water; (2) Substitute a healthy food in place of your *food vice*; (3) Replace sedentary TV time with exercise.

Today presents an opportunity to take an additional step in the direction of a full-time lifestyle of health and fitness. Remember, you are making changes that are creating a permanent positive and healthy lifestyle.

  LESS IS MORE

When it comes to exercising and getting involved in more physical activity, one of the biggest mistakes is to try to do too much too soon. If you are very motivated to lose weight and get fit, you may just want to jump right in and get a gym membership, start going to a kickboxing or other class, as well as begin using all of the muscle-strengthening machines. Unfortunately this gung ho attitude can backfire. There are three risks of trying to overdo it when starting an exercise program—even if you are renewing a past habit of exercising: injury, soreness, and quitting. The downside (the harm) of doing too much too soon outweighs the upside (the benefits). You will be disappointed if all you have to show for your hard work for one day (or even one week) is nothing but soreness or injury. Additionally, if you factor in the changes required to keep up such a demanding pace you are setting yourself up for failure.

So, how do you best avoid jumping in with all cylinders running and risk burning out? You do less. The less-is-more mantra holds true when it comes to exercise. If you do enough to get you into the habit of devoting a thirty-minute segment of time to fitness, you will have a better chance at long-term success. If you don't feel like exercising, then just do what you can. You might find that you will start to do more when you begin just because it starts to feel good.

Goal: Thirty Minutes Daily

I recommend making your first exercise goal to do sustained cardiovascular activity for thirty minutes. What this means is that if you go for a walk outside during your lunch hour, your goal is, at some point over the next few days or weeks, to walk for thirty minutes without stopping. If you can do only five minutes now, that is fine—do five minutes. Gradually build upon your current level of activity until you are able to do thirty minutes.

Cardiovascular exercise focuses on the correct frequency, intensity, and duration of specific techniques. A simple definition of cardiovascular exercise is any exercise that raises your heart rate to a level at which you can still talk but you start to sweat a little. At least twenty minutes of cardiovascular exercise three or four days a week should be enough to maintain a good fitness level.

Any movement is good, even house- or yard work. But if your goal is to lose weight, you will need to do some form of cardiovascular exercise for four or more days a week for thirty to forty-five minutes or longer. The ideal cardiovascular exercise program starts with a five- to ten-minute warm-up, which includes gentle movements that will slightly increase your heart rate. Then, slowly move into twenty or more minutes of a cardiovascular exercise of your choice, such as aerobics, jogging on a treadmill, or walking. Walking is probably the easiest form of exercise to fit into any lifestyle. The convenience of walking makes it ideal—no need for special equipment or memberships. (Of course, before starting this, or any diet and exercise program, consult your physician.)

Because cardiovascular exercise will make a vast improvement in your fitness if you do it each day, the second goal is to work your way up to doing thirty minutes **every day** for six days a week. By the end of one or two months, you should be putting in six days a week (depending on your level of fitness).

Remember, consistency is just as important as actually doing thirty minutes. If you do miss one day, don't beat yourself up, but just think about when and where you will make up the time you were going to exercise. Only the cumulative effects of exercising every day will lead to weight loss, fitness, and a healthy body.

Just as it is not okay to have "just one" when you are trying to get your eating on track and bust these vices, it is also not okay to put off your exercise. Make exercise as important and necessary in your life as getting sleep, because it will make a world of difference. You do not need rest days in between your cardiovascular workout days as you would in between weight-lifting days. Ideally your body should have some sort of cardio movement every day.

 ## COMMON CONCERNS

Most people have certain concerns when it comes to exercise. Some feel self-conscious about the way they look when they go to the gym. Remember, **you are not your body.** In other words, you *have* a body, and if you lost a limb, you'd have less body, but that doesn't mean you'd be any less of the wonderful person that you are. Your weight is something you have but you're doing something about it.

Some people have concerns about time, sweating during the day, the right equipment, the right environment and temperature, and more. The main issue to focus on is figuring out the *how* so you'll never have to worry about the *can't*. Take action and get in your daily physical activity—put yourself in a position of going through the motions if you have to at first. Remember, one step at a time will get you where you want to go.

 Daily Positive Affirmation

I have unlimited confidence in my abilities and myself. I am thankful for the endless opportunities that each day provides. I welcome optimal health into my life!

DAY 20

Actions: (1) Carry a water bottle with you and drink plenty of water; (2) Substitute a healthy food in place of your *food vice*; (3) Replace sedentary TV time with exercise.

Because you are focusing on exercise this week, it's important to find one you can do routinely that is comfortable. If you walk on a treadmill for thirty minutes a day and get into the habit of doing that every day, you will build confidence in yourself and your abilities. You will be eliminating the what-to-do along with the when-to-do-it, and your life will run a lot smoother that way. Having a set time for exercise and a particular exercise to engage in takes away any guesswork and makes you accountable (to yourself) because you will have a time scheduled for your exercise, and you will have the exercise you're going to perform already picked out. Remember, one reason we have an obesity epidemic is because of the difficulty we have changing our daily habits. What better way to change than by keeping things as simple as possible to start.

 MASTER ONE EXERCISE

The purpose of finding one good cardio exercise you like is so that you can *master it.* If you consistently walked for thirty minutes nonstop, you could eventually challenge yourself to more by increasing your speed, or the time in which you walk, or the distance of your walk. Most types of exercise equipment have programmable features that will allow you to monitor your progress and help you know when and how to increase your effort. Machines can be a bit overwhelming at first so keep it simple or ask one of the trainers at the gym to show you how—that's what they are there for.

All of the factors of exercise—time, type of exercise, comfortable workout clothes and shoes—push you to plan ahead. The more you do it, the more it will become part of your daily routine.

Try a few different exercises this first week or take classes such as body pump, step aerobics, or even kickboxing. But by the end of the week choose which *one exercise* you will put your attention and effort toward. After you have *mastered one exercise*—and it won't take as long as you might think—you will have confidence to try other exercises, not to mention other activities that you've wanted to do or try in *any area of your life*. It is always a good idea to change your exercise routine from time to time so that you don't get bored or too comfortable doing the same old thing.

When I say *master*, I don't mean that you'll become an Olympic-class or professional athlete, but I do mean that you will achieve a certain level of confidence and competence while doing the exercise.

Mastering an Exercise *Involves*:

1. Knowledge of the exercise being performed;
2. Familiarity with the uses of any equipment needed;
3. Having the clothes needed for different conditions;
4. Knowing the level of intensity to keep you within your ideal heart range;
5. A set time and location where such exercise is normally performed;
6. Having the ability to perform it at a sustained level for at least thirty minutes;
7. Doing it at least three times a week consistently for twelve weeks.

Approach exercise with the conviction that you are going to *learn the what, when, where, and how* of one enjoyable exercise in order to *master it,* after which you will grow to learn more about other types of exercises and options. In this way you are fully committing yourself to the long-term healthy lifestyle.

 Daily Positive Affirmation
I have unlimited confidence in my abilities and myself. I am thankful for the endless opportunities that each day provides. I welcome optimal health into my life!

DAY 21

Actions: (1) Carry a water bottle with you and drink plenty of water; (2) Substitute a healthy food in place of your *food vice*; (3) Replace sedentary TV time with exercise.

There are plenty of ways to keep track of the progress you have made so far. While weighing yourself is the most common measure used, I think it's the worst measure of all and is something you need to get away from. It's easy to sabotage your efforts by weighing-in too often and becoming discouraged without daily change. Daily weigh-ins don't tell you if you are making progress. How your clothes fit, how you feel, and how well you are sticking to the program are better indicators of success.

 ## WHERE YOU ARE NOW

How do I feel about my progress up to this point?
How does my body feel now compared to when I started?
Can I do more to improve upon what I have done so far?
Is this something I think I can do for the rest of my life?
Do I feel deprived or empowered?

These questions will help you stay on track and hold you accountable for doing the right thing. If you are feeling deprived, you need to list in detail again all of the benefits you're gaining and what you're leaving behind. Possibly you are doing too much too soon and need to scale back so you can make steady and consistent progress. If you feel that you've made any progress at all, that is good. Don't worry whether or not you have *great* results by now. If you feel that you can continue doing what you're doing each day, that's good.

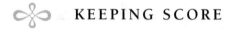 **KEEPING SCORE**

If you like to have a physical measure, or score of your progress thus far, you can complete the following chart:

The number of days I . . .

1. Drank water   _____(21 max)
2. Busted my *food vice*   _____(14 max)
3. Ate healthy substitutes   _____(14 max)
4. Exercised before watching TV   _____(5 max)
5. Completed each day's actions   _____(21 max)

Add up your score and see where you are.

A Total Score of:

65–75: Excellent—you have a strong commitment to good choices and making positive changes;

55–64: Good—one more push and you'll be consistent with your healthy actions;

45–54: Average—you may see results, but you need to increase your consistency and effort;

Below 45: Poor—you need to review your goals and focus; you need to work on mastering only these three actions; go another week or two before moving on.

WEEK 3 SUMMARY

You will achieve positive benefits from exercising if you start making at least thirty minutes of exercise *every day* a part of your on-going lifestyle. *Notice how many of these benefits can reduce your body's mental and physical stress level.*

Regular exercise most likely will . . .

Increase oxygen flow to the body
Get more oxygen to your brain
Elevate your metabolism
Increase your endurance
Improve your cholesterol
Reduce your blood pressure
Decrease triglycerides (fat)
Reduce the risk of dying prematurely
Lessen appearance of aging
Reduce the risk of colon cancer
Improve your attitude
Improve your memory
Reduce anxiety or depression
Promote healing—mind and body

From the Centers for Disease Control and Prevention; http://www.cdc.gov

 ## REWARD YOURSELF

Now that you have completed these first three weeks, why not provide yourself with a reward as reinforcement for your positive actions. Rewards are a great way to condition yourself to continue the healthy and positive actions that will keep you moving toward a healthy weight.

Short-Term Rewards

Visit the local zoo
Get your hair done
Take a long bubble bath
Go on a scenic bike ride
Drive to a new place to take
a walk
Listen to relaxing music and
read a book
Go to see a movie
Rent an old favorite movie
Read a science or astrology
book
Get a pedicure and/or a
manicure
Paint a room in your home a
vibrant new shade
Make curtains for a bright
new look
Buy a new outfit
Buy a new pair of shoes
Teach a child to read
Learn to sew and sew
something
Learn a new craft
Volunteer as a Big Brother or
Big Sister
Bake cookies for the local
firefighters
Sing or perform at a local
nursing home

Do a random act of kindness
Go skydiving (yikes!)
Take a trip to an art museum
Take a walk in the park
Buy a new CD or DVD
Read a book and burn a scented
candle
Buy a new scented candle
Start your own garden
Sign up for a course at a local
college
Contribute time, treasure, or
talent to a charity
Take a computer course
(online?)
Go to the opera or symphony
Send yourself flowers—
anonymously!
Adopt a pet
Study a second language
Go to the library and learn
something new
Take up a new sport
Take up woodworking
Take a painting course
Paint a picture
Go to the park and sketch/
paint
Volunteer for any good cause
Volunteer at a soup kitchen

Milestone-Reaching Rewards

Spend a weekend at a bed-and-breakfast

Have a spa weekend

Have a full day of beauty and a makeover

Buy a new piece of jewelry

Buy a new car

Take an exotic vacation

Visit a historic place

Go skydiving (again? yikes!)

Sing the national anthem (not in the shower)

Rent a horse—and go ride for the day

Take a second honeymoon

Make an exercise room

Buy equipment for a home gym

Put in a new pool (for exercise, of course)

Make a career change

Start your own business

Try something you've never been interested in

Try to overcome a fear you've always had

Buy land in the country

Buy a Harley—and ride for the day

 THIS COMPLETES YOUR FIRST 21 DAYS!

Stick to these three actions from here on out; they are the foundation that you will use to build your healthy new lifestyle:

1. **Plenty of water—eliminate high-sugar drinks**
2. **Vice busting—eliminate unhealthy food(s)**
3. **Regular exercise—reduce or replace TV time**

Ongoing Plan: Weeks 4–12

With twenty-one days behind you, drinking water, eliminating food vices, and exercising should start to become healthy habits. Over the course of the next couple of weeks and beyond the twelve-week mark, you should constantly be focused on *mastering* these three habits.

Over the course of the next nine weeks, you'll keep moving in the direction of a completely fit and healthy lifestyle—**one step each week**. You will see that making one important change at a time and doing it right will be the key to continued success.

When you look around you, you will be able to see physical reminders of your change in lifestyle. Some changes in your environment may include:

1. A case of water bottles (torn open with a few missing)
2. Bananas, or baby carrots, or other healthy snacks used as healthy substitutes
3. Sneakers, and a Walkman or iPod, for exercising
4. Your planner with scheduled time for exercise—in ink!

Your list may be slightly different, but rest assured, you will add more and more as time goes on and these positive health habits become part of your life.

BUILDING A CIRCLE OF HEALTH

I'd like you to visualize the strength that you are creating in your life by making healthy choices. The power that comes with having a well-balanced and healthy life is easier to understand when you live it—you gain a sense of control and confidence from your choices. You become stronger in other areas of your life and even somewhat more secure than you were before.

The confidence comes from knowing that you feel well rounded and balanced—mentally, physically, and even spiritually. Those three can translate to better relationships, improved working conditions, better pay, or even better vacations. You want to strengthen those parts of who **you** are in order that you can grow.

Stepping out of your comfort zone or expanding your reach requires going beyond your *routine thinking* or your *daily routine*. The circle of health is a representation of the strength you gain and the potential areas that are improved as a result of taking full responsibility for living a healthy life.

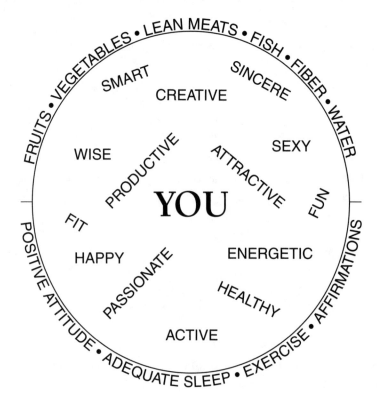

Circle of Health

The actions on the outside of the circle are those that positively influence you. The stronger and more consistent you are with those actions, the stronger your circle of health and the more you can expand in every area of your life.

NEW ACTIONS AND REWARDS

In each of the coming weeks of this plan you will find one new action to perform.

In addition to a weekly action, each week will come with a reward—a way of reinforcing the steps you're taking. This will also be important and very helpful in the game of life as you are earning your way to an even healthier one! You have already been given some ideas of rewards; use them or come up with your own. Either way, **schedule a reward** of some sort for the end of the week so you can look forward to it. I would also suggest that you plan some sort of **bigger reward** for the completion of this twelve-week plan. That should help you feel even more excited to continue on and reach your goal.

There is a saying: "That which you think, you shall become." Keep your thoughts on what is positive and healthy, and soon you will find that the next few weeks bring a tremendous amount of healthy and positive qualities into your life.

 Daily Positive Affirmation
I have unlimited confidence in my abilities and myself. I am thankful for the endless opportunities that each day provides. I welcome optimal health into my life!

cᣟᣞ   **WEEK 4:**

Actions: (1) Adequate Water; (2) Healthy Substitutes; (3) Exercise be-fore TV; (4) Visualize your healthy future.

This week should be used to gain a strong hold on drinking water, eating healthfully, and exercising. Gaining a well-rounded healthy lifestyle starts with emphasizing your commitment to the three actions above. Essentially what you're doing is moving slowly toward your goal of health, and moving away from a life without health. In order to do this more effectively there will be one additional action that you should do this week—**visualizing.**

When you lie down to sleep at night, you want to spend a few min-utes thinking about what your life will look like when you are healthy, happy, fit, and full of energy and excitement. You can imagine your body's being in good shape, looking good, and moving through each day with a new stride in your step. By visualizing each night you are planting the seeds in your brain about what you look like and how you behave. By setting your mind to work while you sleep you are engaging a powerful ally in your quest for a lifetime of good health. In your wak-ing hours your body will need to manifest what your mind is beginning to believe, but your body will take time to adjust and respond to the improvements you have been making.

The Life of a Cell

Your body is constantly changing and working, with each cell doing its part to function as genetically determined and environmentally influ-enced.* Cells have only a particular life span, not unlike yours; some die early because of damage or wear and tear, and some live beyond their normal life span; others are in between. Cells replicate and even-tually become waste as the new ones take over. For example, a typical blood cell will last anywhere from 60 to 120 days. Some tissue in your small intestine may be replaced in a week or less. In the pancreas, it may be a year or more. However, the liver doesn't usually replace its cells unless it shrinks in size (due to damage, possibly); then the cells

*All cell information taken from HHMI.org—Howard Hughes Medical Institute online.

will duplicate (actually divide) to get the liver back to the right size. Some of your skin cells will divide only to keep the skin at a certain thickness.

Each cell is on a different schedule and plan based on its function. Considering the many different rates at which your cells divide and are replaced, your body is going to respond best to repetitive positive healthy habits.

As you begin your changes and start living healthily, let's assume that your body will not fully respond (at least not on the cellular level) to your actions until new cells have replaced old ones. If your body is undergoing a replacement of new cells every few months, you have the opportunity to make even more magnificent changes than you may have realized. Therefore, you must give yourself time when trying to change your body. Genetics and normal function of the cells are going to be a limiting factor that just cannot be altered.

During this fourth week, you should start to see a vast improvement in your energy level from when you started this plan. If you have been following it faithfully, you may find that your mental sharpness has improved as well. If you feel there have not been many physical or mental improvements up to now, don't worry. You should have a daily planner at this point, so that you can keep track of the actions you complete. Evaluate your progress based only on the number of actions you have successfully completed. If you have incorporated these actions into your routine consistently up to now and don't feel you've achieved any results, keep going; you will see change. If you've met or exceeded your goals, be sure you schedule a reward for completing this week's actions.

 KEEPING SCORE

The number of days I . . .

1. Drank water   _____(7 max)
2. Busted my *food vice*   _____(7 max)
3. Ate healthy substitutes   _____(7 max)
4. Exercised before watching TV   _____(5 max)

5. Completed each day's actions _____(7 max)
6. Said my Daily Affirmation _____(7 max)

Add up your score and see where you are.

A Total Score of:

34–40: Excellent—you have a strong commitment to good choices and making positive changes;

27–33: Good—one more push and you'll be consistent with your healthy actions;

21–26: Average—you may see results, but you need to increase your consistency and effort;

Below 20: Poor—you need to review your goals and focus; you need to work on mastering only these four actions; go another week or two before moving on.

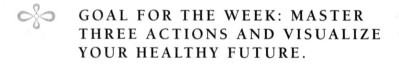 **GOAL FOR THE WEEK: MASTER THREE ACTIONS AND VISUALIZE YOUR HEALTHY FUTURE.**

End of Week Reward: _____

WEEK 5:

Actions: (1) Adequate Water; (2) Healthy Substitutes; (3) Exercise Before TV; (4) Visualize Health; (5) Add a Fruit or Vegetable.

Welcome to Week 5. By now you will have established water as a daily habit and completely busted your *food vice.*

This week you need to add a piece of fruit or a vegetable to whatever you normally eat each day. While you may have added one or the other when busting your *food vice,* this week you need to add another to your daily diet. If you aren't eating healthily during an afternoon snack, or whatever time you reach for something to eat that's not a full meal, then make it a fruit or vegetable. If you already eat healthy snacks (maybe you busted a snack vice), then add a fruit or vegetable to either lunch or dinner.

BENEFITS OF ONE FRUIT OR VEGETABLE

Adding a fruit or vegetable to your daily intake will help you in a number of ways. First, it curbs your appetite. If you have a piece of fruit before lunch you won't be as hungry. If you want a snack in the afternoon, choose a piece of fruit or maybe some baby carrots or a tomato—which will prevent you from craving unhealthy foods. The healthy calories in fruits and vegetables will keep energy levels up and hunger levels down.

By adding another fruit or vegetable to your diet, you will be increasing the amount of water you're consuming. This doesn't count toward your total daily intake, but because most fruits and vegetables have a high water content, you will be providing yourself with a healthy form of water that also happens to be full of vitamins and minerals. The vitamins and/or minerals that are found in most fruits and vegetables are often lacking in most American diets. One dose of a fruit or veggie will help fill this need.

Many fruits and vegetables are high in fiber. Colon cancer is a common illness in our society today, and many experts believe one of the biggest causes is the lack of high-fiber foods in our diet. An extra serving of fruit or vegetable is a great way to start getting the fiber you need. Fiber will help keep your intestines "clean" and keep you regular. Regardless of which expert you agree with—eating more fruits and vegetables will do more good than not having them.

Avoid Hunger

One of the best ways to avoid eating high-calorie snack foods is to eat a piece of fruit or vegetable before the hunger pangs come on. If you can keep from getting hungry, you'll be more likely to succeed in sticking to the plan. In my own experience and my observation of others, when you get to the point of feeling *really* hungry, you are more likely to make poor eating choices. I believe this is due to low sugar levels and your desire to have something immediately to assuage that hunger, but I also think there are probably triggers in your brain that lead you to have what you were used to eating in the past. When you're hungry, you start to focus so much on what to eat that you conjure up images of what you think might taste *really good*. You don't want to put yourself in that situation.

The best way to avoid getting too hungry is to have a piece of fruit or vegetable nearby, especially when you're going to be gone from home all day, or you have a long period between lunch and dinner in the afternoon at work. Having a healthy snack (or two) is fine. You're better off having three bananas than having one doughnut during the day.

I had a client who learned that having one fruit per day was the way to end her daily hunger. Carolyn drank a cup of coffee during the afternoon because she would feel sluggish. This wasn't necessarily a diet vice for her because she drank only one cup and used a low-calorie sweetener. The problem was that she would eat larger portion sizes for her dinner. By having a solid and healthy snack in the middle to late afternoon instead of coffee, she found that her energy level did not experience the same lull *and* she didn't feel as hungry when it was time for dinner. The solution was simple, healthy, and easy.

This week, make plans to have a piece of fruit or vegetable added to your daily diet and get into the habit. It feels extremely good to be eating a healthy food full of water, vitamins, and fiber. These are energy foods—and straight from nature. Be sure you do this week's action at least 80 percent as well as you possibly can and schedule a reward for your time, effort, and success. By the end of this week, exercise should be established as a habit.

 ## KEEPING SCORE

The number of days I . . .

1. Drank water   _____(7 max)
2. Busted my *food vice*   _____(7 max)
3. Ate healthy substitutes   _____(7 max)
4. Exercised before watching TV   _____(5 max)
5. Completed each day's actions   _____(7 max)
6. Said my Daily Affirmation   _____(7 max)

Add up your score and see where you are.

A Total Score of:

34–40: Excellent—you have a strong commitment to good choices and making positive changes
27–33: Good—one more push and you'll be consistent with your healthy actions
21–26: Average—you may see results, but you need to increase your consistency and effort
Below 20: Poor—you need to review your goals and focus; you need to work on mastering only these five actions; go another week or two before moving on

 ## GOAL FOR THE WEEK: ADD A FRUIT OR VEGETABLE TO YOUR DAILY DIET.

End of Week Reward: _____

❦   WEEK 6:

Actions: (1) Adequate Water; (2) Healthy Substitutes; (3) Exercise Before TV; (4) Visualize Health; (5) Add a Fruit/Vegetable; (6) Increase Exercise.

You have come this far and a big "Congratulations" is in order. There may be days that you don't get enough water, exercise, and healthier foods. It happens, but don't let a small setback deter you from your goals. If you said, *"I'm not going to the gym because I'll only get twenty minutes of exercise in,"* go anyway because some exercise is better than none. If you haven't had enough water, be sure you planned ahead to get more the next day.

When you are planning to add a healthy habit to your routine, establish the healthy habit first, then strive to do it to its completion.

If you keep these two points in mind, you won't get down on yourself if you fall short of being thorough with any action during any particular week. Remember, doing the action (making it a habit) is your first priority. **Do it, then worry about doing it exactly right later.**

❦   EXERCISE—VITAL TO HEALTH

This week you should put more emphasis and focus on the exercise that you're doing. You should evaluate your level of health and fitness (see Appendix I), determining if you've made any progress to a higher level. When you started, if you could walk for only five minutes and now you are up to ten minutes, that is an improvement. This is a very individual process, and only you will be able to evaluate how you are feeling and what gains you are realizing. Exercise is one of the most important actions you can take for your health—almost as important as what you eat and drink. The goal for establishing exercise in your routine is to do it at least five days a week. When you reach a frequency of five days and forty-five minutes to an hour each time, you'll be in *very good* shape—it's just a matter of gradual improvements over time. This is an average, so keep in mind that such factors as your job, health conditions, what you're eating, and your genetics all have an influence.

The goal, if you are starting out, is to do mostly cardiovascular or aerobic exercises (like walking, biking, elliptical machine), but eventually you should also be spending time doing muscle-strengthening exercises. If you are not already doing strength-training exercise, you can add that this week. Strength training can be as simple as a rubber band/resistance workout to a weight-lifting session with a trainer at a gym. Just make sure you know how to do it properly and build gradually as you are doing with the cardiovascular exercise. The time you spend exercising should be done performing the recommended exercises for your level (or those recommended to you by a professional).

Your goal this week is to get in at least thirty minutes of exercise for five days this week. There are a couple of things to consider about this time period. First, it's easier (and more effective) to do your thirty minutes all at once. I've been asked if a thirty-minute walk could be split up into two fifteen-minute walks. If you find that you can do thirty minutes *only* if you split it up, by all means do it that way. Eventually, though, you will want to do your minutes all at once. One very good reason—fat burning happens more after your first twenty minutes of continuous exercise. When you start to add muscle strengthening to your routine, you can split up your exercise time if you have to. For this week, your goal is to hit the thirty minutes a day for five days—and plan on it from here on out. Remember that you only apply the actual time that you're exercising toward your 30 minutes—from the moment you start until you're done. Stopping for a five-minute break (for whatever reason) does not count toward your time. Be honest and dedicated to those thirty minutes—they're strictly for you and your health.

With more time dedicated to physical activity, you will either be watching less television or spending more hours exercising while you're watching TV. The rule is to *exercise before or during your TV viewing*. Do that one exercise that you've come to know well and continue to do it more often. You can become an expert on your exercise of choice and how much you're capable of in what amount of time (not your maximum, but what you can comfortably do plus some). Then you can continue to strive for a little bit more speed or distance (and time) in the coming weeks. Don't allow yourself to lay on the couch and watch TV if you haven't yet done your daily exercise—ever!

Focus on Your Target

As you establish good habits and are convinced that progress comes down to whether you are completing daily actions, you should start to become more focused on a weekly target. This is part of the building process that connects what needs to be done now with the result you want to achieve. The visualization process helps, but having a short-term target will bridge the gap between today's actions and the healthy lifestyle that you've been visualizing. Plan ahead for what you want to accomplish for the coming week: set your schedule, buy the necessary groceries, know what times of what days you're going to exercise, and so on. Use achieving these goals as a measure of your progress.

Janet has seen results from vice busting and even more from exercising. She weighed 263 pounds at age forty-seven, and at 5 feet 4 inches, was having difficulty with her energy level and making it through a whole day without a lot of fatigue. Well, after some vice busting—especially giving up television in favor of exercise—she started doing exceptionally well. After she got in the habit of walking, she worked her way up to regular gym visits. Soon after, Janet was down 35 pounds. She went on to lose about 60 pounds and feels that joining a gym was the turning point to getting fit and keeping the weight off. It goes to show you that a little extra effort can go a long way—especially when it's exercise.

Keeping Score

The number of days I . . .

1. Drank water   _____(7 max)
2. Busted my *food vice*   _____(7 max)
3. Ate healthy substitutes   _____(7 max)
4. Exercised before watching TV _____(5 max)
5. Completed each day's actions   _____(7 max)
6. Said my Daily Affirmation   _____(7 max)

Add up your score and see where you are.

A Total Score of:

34–40:   Excellent—you have a strong commitment to good choices and making positive changes

27–33:   Good—one more push and you'll be consistent with your healthy actions

21–26:   Average—you may see results, but you need to increase your consistency and effort

Below 20:   Poor—you need to review your goals and focus; you need to work on mastering only these six actions; go another week or two before moving on

 GOAL FOR THE WEEK: INCREASE THE DAYS/TIME FOR EXERCISE.

End of Week Reward: _____

⚬ **WEEK 7:**

Actions: (1) Adequate Water; (2) Healthy Substitutes; (3) Exercise Before TV; (4) Visualize Health; (5) Add a Fruit/Vegetable; (6) Increase Exercise; (7) Add Fiber.

At this point you should be feeling quite a few positive changes to your overall health. I have seen plenty of people lose at least 10 pounds and many others up to 15 pounds by now. That's only 2 pounds per week, nothing unreasonable or overly dramatic—maybe not impressive enough to get your attention. The fact is this approach makes it easy, doable, and lasting.

This week we take a step to improving your health and even more specifically the health of a very important part of your system: your heart. According to the American Heart Association, cardiovascular (heart and blood vessels) disease ranks as America's number one killer, taking 41 percent of those who die each year. It's been said that too often the first sign of heart problems is a heart attack. Well, besides exercise (and an overall healthy diet), there is one action that you need to do this week and continue to make a part of your ongoing healthy lifestyle: adding fiber to your diet. A diet with an adequate amount of fiber may just help lower high levels of cholesterol, prevent some cancers, control diabetes to some degree, and may prevent gallstones and kidney stones.

⚬ **FIBER—OVERCOMING A DEFICIENCY**

According to the surgeon general, the average American diet gets barely half of the recommended amount of fiber each day.* So what is fiber and why is it so important? Fiber is a substance that your body **cannot digest.** Because you cannot digest it, it is not considered any measurable source of calories. That's right, **fiber = no calories.**

There are two types of fiber: **soluble fiber,** which dissolves in water, and **insoluble,** which does not. Soluble fiber sources include oat

---

*Unless indicated, all fiber and fiber-related information was obtained from the American Heart Association www.americanheart.org.

bran, oatmeal, prunes, beans, peas, rice bran, barley, apples, oranges, peaches, pears, strawberries, and other citrus fruits. **Oats have the highest proportion of soluble fiber of any grain.** Soluble fiber has health benefits, such as helping to lower cholesterol, relieving constipation, and even relieving hemorrhoids. It has a positive influence in the prevention of heart disease by helping to control cholesterol and triglyceride levels. Adequate fiber can also help regulate blood sugar levels, which is important in avoiding diabetes. Many experts agree that a diet with adequate amounts of fiber may help prevent colon cancer. (Fiber benefits taken from http://yourmedicalsource.com.)

Insoluble fiber does not dissolve in water. Insoluble fiber sources include whole wheat breads, wheat cereals, wheat bran, popcorn, brown rice, rye, barley, carrots, Brussels sprouts, turnips, cauliflower, and apple skin (the rest of the apple is *soluble*). Insoluble fiber doesn't have the same benefits as soluble but seems to be especially important to the normal functioning of the bowel. This type bulks up waste and moves it through the bowels more efficiently. According to the Johns Hopkins Medical Center (www.jhbmc.jhu.edu), "Fiber is a [dieters'] dream since fibers called cellulose and hemicellulose take up space in the stomach, making us feel full, therefore food intake is less." What that means is you can use a fiber-rich food or drink to curb your appetite without getting the calories (only so often, **not** three times per day).

You can increase the fiber in your diet by adding another fruit or vegetable or salad to your daily intake or you can follow my suggestion below.

Buy some bran cereal that is low in carbohydrates yet high in fiber. Watch out for extra and unnecessary sugars when getting bran cereal—Kellogg's makes one called All-Bran that's good (with a low carb option) and Kashi also makes a good one. Then pick up some wheat germ and milled flaxseed. Wheat germ (I use *Mother's* brand) contains vitamin E, some B vitamins, zinc, and some minerals, and is believed to help colon function, nourish the skin, lower cholesterol, and boost the immune system. The milled flaxseed is believed to have similar benefits—assists with colon function, helps lower cholesterol, provides a source of *good* fats (omega-3 fatty acids), and is a good soluble fiber (with some insoluble too).

Put a small portion (a half cup or less) of your *bran cereal* in a bowl. Add one teaspoonful of *milled flaxseed* and one tablespoonful of *wheat germ*. Add skim milk (or soy milk with low carbs) and enjoy. You'll be getting a good source of fiber and nutrition without too many calories! Do this once a day, as part of a meal or snack.

SOME SOURCES OF FIBER

Soluble		Insoluble Fiber		
Oatmeal	Legumes:	Whole	Brown rice	Carrots
Oat bran	Dried peas	grains	Cereals	Cucumbers
Nuts and seeds	Beans, Lentils	Whole	Wheat bran	Zucchini
Apples	Strawberries	wheat	Seeds	Celery
Pears	Blueberries	breads	Whole wheat	Tomatoes
		Barley	couscous	

From www.hsph.harvard.edu/nutritionsource/fiber.html

Fruits; Serving size; Total fiber (g)	Grains, cereal, pasta; Serving size; Total fiber (g)
Pear 1 medium 5.1	Spaghetti, whole-wheat 1 cup 6.3
Figs, dried 2 medium 3.7	Bran flakes ¾ cup 5.3
Blueberries 1 cup 3.5	Oatmeal 1 cup 4.0
Apple, with skin 1 medium 3.3	Bread, rye 1 slice 1.9
Peaches, dried 3 halves 3.3	Bread, whole-wheat 1 slice 1.9
Orange 1 medium 3.1	Bread, mixed-grain 1 slice 1.7
Strawberries 1 cup 3.0	Bread, cracked-wheat 1 slice 1.4
Apricots, dried 10 halves 2.6	
Raisins 1.5-ounce box 1.6	

Legumes, nuts, seeds; Serving size; Total Fiber (g)	Vegetables; Serving size; Total fiber (g)
Lentils 1 cup 15.6	Peas 1 cup 8.8
Black beans 1 cup 15.0	Artichoke, cooked 1 medium 6.5
Baked beans, canned 1 cup 13.9	Brussels sprouts 1 cup 6.4
Lima beans 1 cup 13.2	Turnip greens, boiled 1 cup 5.0
Almonds 24 nuts 3.3	Potato, baked with skin 1 medium 4.4
Pistachio nuts 47 nuts 2.9	Corn 1 cup 4.2
Peanuts 28 nuts 2.3	Popcorn, air-popped 3 cups 3.6
Cashews 18 nuts 0.9	Tomato paste ¼ cup 3.0
	Carrot 1 medium 1.8

From Mayo Clinic: www.mayoclinic.com

Citrucel and **Metamucil** are good forms of insoluble fiber that can be consumed once a day or as directed by your doctor.

Juice Plus+® provides whole-food-based nutrition from seventeen fruits, vegetables, and grains—plus fiber blends—in convenient capsule form. It helps provide the variety of antioxidants and phytochemicals that only whole foods offer.

Adding fiber to your diet may be one of the most important actions you can do to change your health dramatically in the short term. It may also keep you from being part of an alarming statistic of people who have heart and artery problems that turn into heart attacks or strokes.

Note: A large increase in fiber over a short period of time may result in bloating, diarrhea, gas, and general discomfort. It is important to add fiber *gradually* over a period of time (three weeks) to avoid abdominal problems.

Keeping Score

The number of days I . . .

1. Drank water   _____(7 max)
2. Busted my *food vice*   _____(7 max)
3. Ate healthy substitutes   _____(7 max)
4. Exercised before watching TV   _____(5 max)
5. Completed each day's actions   _____(7 max)
6. Said my Daily Affirmation   _____(7 max)

Add up your score and see where you are.

A Total Score of:

34–40:   Excellent—you have a strong commitment to good choices and making positive changes

27–33:   Good—one more push and you'll be consistent with your healthy actions

21–26:   Average—you may see results, but you need to increase your consistency and effort

Below 20: Poor—you need to review your goals and focus; you need to work on mastering only these seven actions; go another week or two before moving on

 GOAL FOR THE WEEK: ADD FIBER TO YOUR DIET.

End of Week Reward: _____

WEEK 8:

Actions: (1) Adequate Water; (2) Healthy Substitutes; (3) Exercise Before TV; (4) Visualize Health; (5) Add a Fruit/Vegetable; (6) Increase Exercise; (7) Add Fiber; (8) Clean Your Home.

As the building process continues, you're growing toward a life you are visualizing that is complete with healthy thoughts, actions, body, mind, and spirit.

If you have made the commitment to do the actions outlined up to this point, you should be feeling a sense of empowerment and control. Don't stop to celebrate by letting up, but do take the time to have a reward scheduled for the end of each week—but only if you've completed your goals for the week. You decide what completing them is: 70 percent, 80 percent, or is it adhering to your plan 100 percent? I'm not going to set a number for you; if you feel good about your progress, then do what you have planned at the end of each week. Even the smallest amount of improvement each week will add up to bigger changes in your life over time—take this journey at the pace that is right for you.

GET YOUR HOUSE IN ORDER

This week we're going to shift the focus to your surroundings. One of the things I have noticed over the years is how many people too often approach weight loss and dieting as being separate from normal daily living. As we've established by now, you can't be on a diet part-time, lose some weight, and go back to the way things were. You absolutely should not. In order for you to continue progressively moving toward a healthy lifestyle, let's look at your surroundings, mainly your home.

The first and most obvious place to start is your kitchen. How many snacks, unhealthy treats, high-sugar foods are in your kitchen? Does the life that you've been visualizing include all of those? Look to be sure that you aren't stashing items that you don't need or that don't belong in your life anymore.

The kitchen is the place where, if tempted by unhealthy foods, you're most likely to be consuming unhealthy calories.

Toss out the unhealthy foods and drinks and be sure that healthier foods are available and handy. Fresh fruit in a bowl on the table, high-fiber cereals in the pantry, snack-size carrots or other vegetables in the refrigerator, sliced and ready for eating. Be sure to wash your hands before handling food—it is the first defense in preventing sickness.

Healthy = Clean

If you are going to work toward a healthy and fit lifestyle, your home should be suitable for someone who *is healthy and fit*. Once you've tackled the cleaning and organizing, you will have a clean and organized kitchen. You'll feel a renewed sense of energy and a greater affinity with your surroundings, and that's *good* energy. I'd also like to point out that you may get the feeling of a fresh start (like a do-over) where from here on out you're moving only in the direction of health and leaving behind that other lifestyle. Focus on cleaning and organizing your home this week, in addition to the other actions—*and don't forget to schedule a reward.*

Keeping Score

The number of days I . . .

1. Drank water   _____(7 max)
2. Busted my *food vice*   _____(7 max)
3. Ate healthy substitutes   _____(7 max)
4. Exercised before watching TV   _____(5 max)
5. Completed each day's actions   _____(7 max)
6. Said my Daily Affirmation   _____(7 max)

Add up your score and see where you are.

A Total Score of:

34–40: Excellent—you have a strong commitment to good choices and making positive changes

27–33: Good—one more push and you'll be consistent with your healthy actions

21–26: Average—you may see results, but you need to increase your consistency and effort

Below 20: Poor—you need to review your goals and focus; you need to work on mastering only these eight actions; go another week or two before moving on

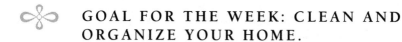 **GOAL FOR THE WEEK: CLEAN AND ORGANIZE YOUR HOME.**

End of Week Reward: _____

c⧉o   **WEEK 9:**

Actions: (1) Adequate Water; (2) Healthy Substitutes; (3) Exercise Before TV; (4) Visualize Health; (5) Add a Fruit/Vegetable; (6) Increase Exercise; (7) Add Fiber; (8) Clean Your Home; (9) Add a Daily Supplement.

I'd like you to take the time at this point to do a quick self-evaluation to determine your progress. Please write down the answers to your questions in enough detail so that it will reinforce what you're doing or let you know that some things need more work. I would suggest writing the positive benefits you've experienced in your daily planner so you can reflect on them throughout the day (and add to them or put down ideas on how to improve things).

> **How do I feel about my progress up to this point?**
> **How does my body feel now compared to when I started?**
> **Can I do more to improve upon what I have done so far?**
> **Is this something I think I can do for the rest of my life?**
> **Do I feel deprived or empowered?**

You'll notice that one question still asks you to do a comparison to when you started. As you get ten, eleven, or even twelve weeks into this plan, it may seem a bit ridiculous to compare your progress to your starting point so long ago. Actually, I think it's good to do that so you can keep the overall big picture in mind.

c⧉o   **ADDING ANTIOXIDANT SUPPLEMENTS**

Our environment is much different from that of a century ago. It is subjected to more contaminants, wastes, fumes, gases, and other forms of pollution and toxins now than at any other time in history. There is no doubt that unless we change our course, society as a whole will be faced with an alarming pollution problem. The problem affects the quality of the air we breathe and the quality of the soil used to grow the foods we eat. Pollutants can have a negative impact on our heart, lungs, digestive system, and our reproductive organs. The air, soil, and water quality all influence our overall health (another reason to complete the goal of Week 8). In fact, as reported by the American Association on Mental Retardation (AAMR), approximately 80,000 new synthetic chemicals have been approved for use since World War II, and for the 15,000 most commonly found chemicals today, the vast majority have not been tested individually for human health impacts. This problem is right in front of our faces every day. We can help our own situation, even if we can't immediately change the environment.

You've heard the saying "An ounce of prevention is worth a pound of cure." The ounce of prevention is nutritional supplements. This week's step of taking nutritional supplements will help prevent health problems that can develop as a result of these pollutants that we're all exposed to.

In nutritional terms, we can define a supplement as *a substance that is taken to complete a nutritional need.* The environmental impact seems clear but it's also important to take a look at how our bodies operate and use the nutrition that we gain from food.

Free Radicals

Free radicals are caused by many factors, such as radiation from the sun or X-rays, automobile exhaust, cigarette smoke, alcohol, saturated fat, stress, and chemicals found in foods, water, and air.

Free radicals can cause damage to cell walls, certain cell structures, and genetic material within the cells, leading to aging, arthritis, various cancers, heart disease, cataracts, autoimmune diseases, Alzheimer's, and Parkinson's. So it is important to add antioxidants to your daily diet to reduce the circulating free radicals in your body.

While antioxidants come from fruits and vegetables, it isn't likely that the typical American diet can supply all that we need for ideal health. Some people turn to traditional vitamin supplements but individual vitamins or multivitamins do not supply the thousands of antioxidants and other phytonutrients missing in their diets. In fact, our bodies are genetically programmed to require small amounts of over 12,000 nutrients (including vitamins) working synergistically in a perfect combination found only in fruits and vegetables.

Some research shows that traditional vitamin supplements may even be harmful in large amounts. The reason is because Americans do not have vitamin deficiencies, but instead have whole food deficiencies. We are especially lacking in fruits and vegetables with their thousands of phytonutrients.

ANTIOXIDANTS: SOURCES OF FREE RADICAL FIGHTERS

Food Sources

Carrots	Red grapes	Red kidney beans
Lemons	Raspberries	Black beans
Oranges	Cranberries	Artichokes
Apples	Strawberries	Pecans
Blueberries	Plums	Russet potatoes

From WebMD: http://my.webmd.com/content/article/89/100138.htm

Recommended Supplements

Juice Plus + complete ®
Juice Plus +® Garden, Orchard, and Vineyard Capsules

Start supplementing your diet with enough antioxidants to fight free radicals. You might find that a complete vitamin *and* mineral supplement is the best way to go. Be sure to start supplementing this week *and* plan on doing it every day.

Keeping Score

The number of days I . . .

1. Drank water   _____(7 max)
2. Busted my *food vice*   _____(7 max)
3. Ate healthy substitutes   _____(7 max)
4. Exercised before watching TV   _____(5 max)
5. Completed each day's actions   _____(7 max)
6. Said my Daily Affirmation   _____(7 max)

Add up your score and see where you are.

A Total Score of:

34–40:   Excellent—you have a strong commitment to good choices and making positive changes

27–33:   Good—one more push and you'll be consistent with your healthy actions

21–26:   Average—you may see results, but you need to increase your consistency and effort

Below 20: Poor—you need to review your goals and focus; you need to work on mastering only these nine actions; go another week or two before moving on

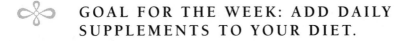 **GOAL FOR THE WEEK: ADD DAILY SUPPLEMENTS TO YOUR DIET.**

End of Week Reward: _____

⧖   **WEEK 10:**

Actions: (1) Adequate Water; (2) Healthy Substitutes; (3) Exercise Before TV; (4) Visualize Health; (5) Add a Fruit/Vegetable; (6) Increase Exercise; (7) Add Fiber; (8) Clean Your Home; (9) Supplements; (10) Eat a Healthy Breakfast.

This week let's take another look at fiber and supplements. The recommended fiber sources are good for your overall health as described, but did you know that flaxseed is also a good *fighter* of free radicals? How's that for a bonus? One thing to keep in mind: *give yourself time* when it comes to noticing the effects of supplementing your diet. In fact, some effects are not even noticeable. Your actions today could be preventing a disease years from now. Continue to build on the actions you've taken so far.

⧖   **BREAKFAST *FOR* CHAMPIONS**

This week it's time to start paying closer attention to what you're eating for breakfast. You may already be eating a healthy breakfast and that's great. It's often a natural progression without any of my coaching. Don't worry if you are not, this is the week to start.

You've probably heard that breakfast is the most important meal of the day. According to a Harvard Medical School study* of more than 3,500 adults, those who ate breakfast every day were a third *less likely to be obese* compared to those who skipped it.

The study also determined that those who had breakfast were half as likely to have blood sugar problems, which increase the risk of developing diabetes or high cholesterol—both are a risk factor of heart disease. Dr. Periera, who headed the study, said that it appears that breakfast first thing in the morning may help stabilize blood sugar levels, which regulate appetite and energy.

Eating breakfast supports the *avoid hunger* recommendation that I

---

*These findings were presented at the American Heart Association's 2003 annual conference.

gave you on Week 5. If you miss breakfast, you're more likely to get to work and overeat on the unhealthy foods there or that you pick up on the way because you're *really* hungry. You wouldn't be in that predicament if you had something to eat before you left the house. Even if you are a stay-at-home mom, you don't want to wait until your hunger hits a high before you eat.

In a study published in the April 1999 *Journal of the American College of Nutrition,* breakfast eaters had lower cholesterol and got more vitamins and minerals than those who did not eat breakfast or those who did not eat a *hearty breakfast* (defined as *at least* one-quarter of the daily recommended calories). Results from a Georgian Centenarian Study found that those who lived to be 100 years old consumed breakfast more regularly throughout their lifetime than the average person. The November 1999 issue of the *International Journal of Food Science and Nutrition* reported that people who eat breakfast feel sharper mentally and better physically throughout the day than those who don't.

I eat two or three breakfast foods more regularly than others. I suggest that you find a couple of breakfast choices that you like and stick with those for a while. That way you're not running out to buy all kinds of groceries for a different breakfast every morning. And you're not putting too much focus on *food.* Focus on getting good nutrition and move on to getting other things done for the day. You will also see that eating breakfast is the easiest way to get your fiber, based on the selection of recipes. You don't need to necessarily double up on your fiber intake, but you will want to be sure that you have a well-balanced meal if you are going to get your added fiber intake with breakfast. This is also a good time to have another piece of fruit for the day. See Appendix II, the recipe section, for suggestions, page 179.

Keeping Score

The number of days I . . .

1. Drank water   _____(7 max)
2. Busted my *food vice*   _____(7 max)
3. Ate healthy substitutes   _____(7 max)
4. Exercised before watching TV   _____(5 max)

5. Completed each day's actions   _____(7 max)

6. Said my Daily Affirmation   _____(7 max)

Add up your score and see where you are.

A Total Score of:

34–40:   Excellent—you have a strong commitment to good choices and making positive changes

27–33:   Good—one more push and you'll be consistent with your healthy actions

21–26:   Average—you may see results, but you need to increase your consistency and effort

Below 20: Poor—you need to review your goals and focus; you need to work on mastering only these ten actions; go another week or two before moving on

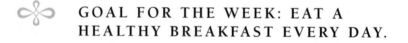 **GOAL FOR THE WEEK: EAT A HEALTHY BREAKFAST EVERY DAY.**

End of Week Reward: _____

WEEK 11:

Actions: (1) Adequate Water; (2) Healthy Substitutes; (3) Exercise Before TV; (4) Visualize Health; (5) Add a Fruit/Vegetable; (6) Increase Exercise; (7) Add Fiber; (8) Clean Home; (9) Supplements; (10) Eat a Healthy Breakfast; (11) Eat a Healthy Lunch.

Although you are nearing the completion of twelve weeks and maybe even your weight loss goal, there is an important lesson about completing what you started. A Chinese proverb says, "When you are 95 percent of the way to your goal, you have only put in 50 percent of the effort needed." This means it may get harder to reach your goal the closer you get.

Surprisingly, most people throw in the towel at the five-yard line of life when they are just pushing past that last struggle, that last hurdle, that last steep climb near the top that would allow them to realize a major goal—the turning point where major results are seen and the joy and pleasure from the dedication comes through.

There is one thing that I can guarantee you: *If you stop putting forth the effort to lose weight and get fit and healthy, you won't lose weight and be fit.* You'll never know if your goal was just one more play or a few more yards. So keep pushing on one "play" at a time.

 A HEALTHY LUNCH

A healthy lunch is the goal of Week 11. When you began to bust your fast-food diet vice, you may have already started eating a healthy lunch—or at least some version of one. If you have, then apply the same principle toward having a healthy snack. The importance for most people of eating a healthy lunch applies to a healthy snack—and that is food that won't slow you down.

For those of us who normally wake up between 6 and 8 a.m., and work (or not) until 5 p.m., lunch comes about noon. This meal fills two important needs. The first is that whatever we're eating provides us with proper nutrition and calories, and the second is that it supports a high energy level for the rest of the day. This may sound like a plea for carbohydrates of some sort and it may be—if you pour concrete all day.

There just aren't too many jobs that require a high-carbohydrate lunch these days, so I don't recommend it unless you have one of them.

Bring It with You

If you work at a job outside your home, you will do yourself a world of good by **packing your own lunch.** This is the only way to definitively know that what you'll be eating is healthy. If you've been working on better snacks, you'll be packing a snack anyway, so you might as well put your lunch with it. Your snack being the extra banana, apple, or whatever works for you. Bringing your lunch allows you to eat some of it during your lunch break and save some for later. You may find that eating half now and half later keeps you from feeling too full and/or being too hungry. Also, you won't be tempted into thinking that you'll just get something healthier when the time comes, only to find out that the gang wants pizza this afternoon.

If you have kids, the latest research suggests that the best way to prevent them from becoming overweight is to be sure they eat a healthy lunch and the best way is to pack it for them. After all, if you're putting a few dollars in their pocket, do you really expect them to select the healthiest food and drink?

Regardless of where you work or what you do, though, you will want to eat light. The most common and best choice for lunch (and dinner) is a salad. There are many ways to make a salad, and just as many that are healthy. You will find quite a few salad choices in Appendix II: Quick and Healthy Recipes (page 179). A salad allows you to get lots of tasty, healthy nutrition, while not slowing you down the way a burger and fries would do. A few folks have told me a salad takes some time and is a bit inconvenient, but it doesn't have to be. Plenty of things can go into a salad that, although perishable, will stay good for most of the day—mushrooms, onions, tomatoes, and artichoke hearts. I like to put grilled chicken with it for the added protein. If you don't think you can make that work, there are other choices. A grilled chicken sandwich with tomatoes, lettuce, and other vegetables is a healthy way to go. Always leave out the potato chips and high-calorie desserts. You'll also find that a good, healthy sandwich is the right choice for the high-energy meal that you need. If you don't have a refrigerator at work, bring a cooler or insulated bag with ice to ensure freshness.

When eating out, remember that you are the one paying for the food and it is okay to specify that you want healthy fare. Grilled meats and fish are always good options; also ask for no sauce or sauce on the side. Beware of hidden calories on items such as grilled vegetables, which many chefs brush with oil to give a better appearance. Tell your server exactly what you want and do not be embarrassed if your needs are off the menu. Your health has to be your biggest concern, not the feelings of the chef—or what your meal companion might think. One other tip is to call ahead to where you are dining and ask them what the healthiest meal they offer is or what they could do to accommodate you, and place your order then. That way you won't have to worry about feeling uncomfortable when ordering at the table.

Focus this week on eating a healthy lunch every day. It can mean the difference between an extremely productive afternoon and an unproductive sluggish one. Be sure to schedule a reward for the end of the week as your incentive to stick to your healthy actions this week.

Keeping Score

The number of days I . . .

1. Drank water	_____(7 max)
2. Busted my *food vice*	_____(7 max)
3. Ate healthy substitutes	_____(7 max)
4. Exercised before watching TV	_____(5 max)
5. Completed each day's actions	_____(7 max)
6. Said my Daily Affirmation	_____(7 max)

Add up your score and see where you are.

A Total Score of:

34–40:   Excellent—you have a strong commitment to good choices and making positive changes

27–33:   Good—one more push and you'll be consistent with your healthy actions

21–26:   Average—you may see results, but you need to increase your consistency and effort

Below 20: Poor—you need to review your goals and focus; you need to . work on mastering only these eleven actions; go another week or two before moving on

     GOAL FOR THE WEEK: EAT A HEALTHY LUNCH EVERY DAY.

End of Week Reward: _____

WEEK 12:

Actions: (1) Adequate Water; (2) Healthy Substitutes; (3) Exercise Before TV; (4) Visualize Health; (5) Add a Fruit/Vegetable; (6) Increase Exercise; (7) Add Fiber; (8) Clean Home; (9) Supplements; (10) Eat a Healthy Breakfast (11) Eat a Healthy Lunch; (12) Eat a Healthy Dinner.

As you enter this final week of the *vice-busting diet plan*, I'm sure you've anticipated what this week has in store for you—that's right, a healthy dinner. The final step toward building a lifestyle of health and fitness, although *not* the least important, is to put your focus on what should be your last meal of the day.

For too many people, dinner comes at a time when their hunger is reaching a peak. You've worked all day and gone most of the afternoon without much in the way of nutrition. While we've covered the importance of not letting yourself get hungry, one of the hardest things to do is plan your dinner—especially when you and/or your spouse work away from home—and it may be tempting to grab something on the way back.

If you have gone too long without food, it usually leads to dinner's being the biggest meal of the day. Unfortunately, having your biggest meal at this time gives you too much opportunity to consume too many calories and therefore put on more weight. The family time you might have is terrific, but the calories ingested are not. Like so many Americans, you may not be having a big sit-down dinner because of our now fast-paced society, but you still may be eating too much of the wrong foods at the wrong time.

DINNER AT THE RIGHT TIME

The next biggest issue with dinner tends to be *eating too late* or too close to when you go to sleep. You don't want to put a whole bunch of calories in your system only to sit or lie down. Another cause for the prevalence of late evening (over-?) eating is television. Evening is when people watch the most TV—and that means snacks are likely to come with it.

If you've been doing your daily exercises, I'm guessing that you may be doing them (or it) first thing after work. If you are exercising after work, you're probably postponing your dinner. This can be good but also risky.

Exercise can make you hungry, and that can lead to a greater likelihood of overeating. To get your exercise in yet avoid the consequences of overeating, you should be having a snack and some water by the time you're ready to leave work. Be sure your snack will provide energy for whatever exercise you're doing. If you're walking for thirty minutes, then maybe just a banana; if you're doing twenty minutes of jogging followed by thirty minutes of muscle strengthening, maybe have a light protein shake with fruit.

Now, after you've exercised you're going to eat when you get home, but you're not going to sit down to a traditional meal of meat, potatoes, vegetables, bread, and so on because you don't ever want to be consuming all that food at once anymore. **Dinner needs to become the least important of all three meals.** Because you've had a postwork snack, make your postworkout snack one for recovery and rebuilding from exercise: a high-protein, no-fat, low-carb shake or food. You won't need extra energy to sleep and you don't want the calories unless you're trying to gain weight. If you don't exercise after work you can still employ the same principle of a split dinner. Have a little something healthier before heading home and don't load up on calories at the dinner table.

As dinner becomes the least important, breakfast is the most important. Starting your day with good nutrition will set the stage for how productive you are, how much energy you have, and how sharp your mind will be. Lunch will be a continuation of that energy level and sharpness, while dinner needs to be a lighter meal that is for recovery—giving your muscles and tissues (including your brain) some necessary nutrition so that you can wind down and relax. You can eat two or three more times—once in the afternoon, once before exercise, and one light snack at least an hour (maybe two) before bed. You're up to eating six times a day! Many experts agree that breaking up your food intake into six smaller meals is better than eating three larger ones.

Four Aspects of a Good Diet

1. Breakfast is the most important meal of the day—then lunch, then dinner;
2. Healthy snacks keep energy levels high and blood sugar levels from getting low;
3. Nutrition throughout the day (up to six times) keeps you ready for any task;
4. You'll have more energy and make a quicker recovery— especially from exercising.

Start your day right, build on your first healthy meal with a healthy, energy-rich lunch, followed by a snack in the afternoon and even one before you exercise. Be sure to reward yourself this week.

Keeping Score

The number of days I . . .

1. Drank water   _____(7 max)
2. Busted my *food vice*   _____(7 max)
3. Ate healthy substitutes   _____(7 max)
4. Exercised before watching TV   _____(5 max)
5. Completed each day's actions   _____(7 max)
6. Said my Daily Affirmation   _____(7 max)

Add up your score and see where you are.

A Total Score of:

34–40: Excellent—you have a strong commitment to good choices and making positive changes

27–33: Good—one more push and you'll be consistent with your healthy actions

21–26: Average—you may see results, but you need to increase your consistency and effort

Below 20: Poor—you need to review your goals and focus; you need to work on mastering only these twelve actions; go another week or two before moving on.

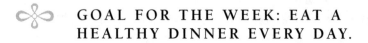 **GOAL FOR THE WEEK: EAT A HEALTHY DINNER EVERY DAY.**

End of Week Reward: _____

A 12-WEEK REVIEW

I hope you are as excited as I am at the prospect of your completing twelve weeks of healthy changes on your way to a lifestyle of health and fitness. First, congratulations for coming this far.

If you feel as if you have fallen short on some of your actions, don't despair. You don't have to do every action to lose weight, because making these changes isn't only about losing weight—it's about successfully keeping it off. The only way to do that is to choose a lifestyle of health and fitness, which means working on developing healthy habits. If you can engage in healthy habits *most* of the time, you will find that you'll no longer have to diet and you'll no longer have problems with major weight fluctuations.

We all make mistakes, have setbacks, and even get off the right track—sometimes without even knowing it until the unwanted effect of our actions happens. Most of the time, it's in the form of added weight. It happens, and it may have happened to you during the last twelve weeks. But by following the bare minimum of actions outlined, you won't see major weight fluctuations. If you embrace the philosophy of this plan—keeping things simple and sticking to the basics—you won't need to wonder or worry about what to do if and when you start to get off track.

These questions will help you determine if what you are doing can be sustained as part of your desire for a healthy and fit lifestyle. Also, please notice the slight change to the third question, since we've covered the actions necessary for a complete and well-rounded healthy lifestyle.

How do I feel about my progress up to this point?
How does my body feel now compared to when I started?
Can I continue doing what I'm doing?
Is this something I think I can do for the rest of my life?
Do I feel deprived or empowered?

Answer these questions positively and you'll feel the confidence to continue your pursuit of health and fitness. If you don't feel you can honestly answer each one positively, continue doing the actions you *can* do now, and work to acquire the rest of them—one at a time.

✤ THE VICE-BUSTING DIET

Summary

Week 1: *BUST* your soft drink diet vice—goal: consume water 90 percent of time

Week 2: *BUST* your fast-food diet vice—goal: replace vice with a healthy substitute

Week 3: *BUST* your television vice—goal: exercise thirty minutes a day three days a week

Week 4: Goal—Master the first three actions; visualize a healthy future—daily

Week 5: Goal—Fruit or Vegetable: add one to your daily diet

Week 6: Goal—Exercise: Increase the days and/or time for exercise

Week 7: Goal—Fiber: Increase your daily fiber intake

Week 8: Goal—Organize: clean and organize your kitchen and home

Week 9: Goal—Supplements: add a daily supplement to fight free radicals

Week 10: Goal—Breakfast: eat a healthy and hearty breakfast each day

Week 11: Goal—Lunch: eat a healthy and high-energy lunch every day

Week 12: Goal—Dinner: eat a healthy dinner—not a large one—each day

Chapter 6

Staying on Track for Greater Health and Fitness

The biggest factor when it comes to completing any goal is your motivation. If you don't have enough reasons why you want to achieve the goal of weight loss, your chances of losing weight decrease, and your chances of losing weight *and* living a healthy lifestyle get close to zero. If you become content or satisfied along the way to what would be considered an excellent physique, you may find yourself staying there—or worse, *stuck there*.

With a little bit of success many of us slip into a comfortable zone and get content, which is not necessarily a good thing when we're capable of so much more. Contentment can breed laziness. And laziness will eventually breed bad habits. So regardless of how well you've done up to this point, don't believe for a minute that it's okay to relax and enjoy how smart you are and how in control you are, because as soon as that happens you're headed for a fall off the wagon. It happened to me more times than I remember and it has to countless others—it's human nature.

What is it that will *keep* you motivated as you move on and continue to develop healthy habits, or as you live those healthy habits day-to-day *for the rest of your life*? How can you help support your own commitment to health every day when unhealthy choices seem to be all around?

As you go forward here are some tips/suggestions for better health and fitness:

- Stock water bottles and water filters for spouts and pitchers
- Drink 8 ounces of water first thing in the morning
- Find healthy foods to substitute in place of unhealthy ones
- Perform crunches (short sit-ups) for ninety seconds each morning
- Plan to bring lunch and snacks instead of buying
- Avoid restaurants unless for special occasions
- Eat a piece of fruit with breakfast and *before* lunch
- Use breakfast as a time to get needed fiber
- Eat plain oatmeal often—add milled flaxseed oil and wheat germ
- Use lunch as a time to get vegetables by having a salad
- Schedule exercise at a consistent time each day
- Have an exercise partner so you can both encourage each other
- Do thirty minutes of sustained aerobic exercise six days per week
- Use muscle-strengthening exercises three days per week
- Exercise during, or instead of, watching television
- Plan to do something physical instead of watching television
- Make healthy pastimes part of life—reading magazines, activities, trips, hobbies
- Involve your family with your healthy choices
- Focus on living a balanced lifestyle
- Visualize, each day, a life full of health and happiness—say the daily affirmations
- Live a healthy and fit lifestyle for the rest and best of your life

Keep a **POSITIVE MENTAL ATTITUDE** by **using daily affirmations**.

SCHEDULE TIME TO RELAX AND RECOVER

We've all heard that *"life is too short . . ."* and the rest of that saying you can complete with any number of choices. We really don't need to, and shouldn't be, using our most valuable commodity—time—for doing nothing. I do think that overall we tend to mix rest, relaxation, and breaks throughout the day and that the mere action of relaxing or resting is given little or no importance. Relaxing is equally important when it comes to the items on your daily schedule. How great to have time to yourself to focus on nothing but being completely at ease and quiet.

Many of us may be busy doing something we may *not* enjoy (or at least *not* find joy in doing) and would rather be doing something else. That may lead to doing . . . well . . . nothing, more often than necessary. First *find joy* in whatever you're doing—your job, career, chores, and so on—and find ways to do them better, smarter, or more efficiently. The second thing, of course, is to set aside a time to relax (or meditate or pray or just be alone and quiet). This is time to be used to reflect on what's good about your life *right now* and that will also give you some mental (and physical) recovery from life's stresses.

If you've got a specified time for doing nothing but relaxing, the time you're not relaxing will give you more reason and motivation to do a better job, put in more effort, or just get the job (or tasks, projects, and so on) done faster. Let's face it, you can't do a job, task, or project and rest and relax at the same time. Why not schedule the time to relax so that you can focus on the job at hand? I'm suggesting that when you've got time in your day that will be set aside specifically for resting your mind and body you can push forward to get your scheduled tasks for the day finished even when you feel like taking a break.

Look at your day—today—and count the minutes where you find yourself doing nothing but relaxing and clearing your mind. No phone, television, music, conversation, or noise (if possible)—just the sound of silence. There are plenty of books written on this subject and most of them cover it under the topic of meditation. Call it what you like, but being on the go constantly—mentally or physically—is not the way of optimal health. Set aside fifteen minutes of time before you fall asleep. Use the time to think about all that is good in your life, and all the things that you're making better. You can even use the suggested positive affirmations to start out. Follow through with this—you'll be glad you did.

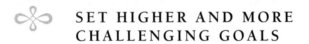

SET HIGHER AND MORE CHALLENGING GOALS

You can lose momentum if you're not putting yourself to greater tests and challenges. There are so many things that you may be capable of doing that maybe you just haven't considered. By setting higher and more challenging goals for yourself, you will keep your life interesting, fun, and adventurous. I think there is some sort of preconceived notion that challenges and goals have to be hard work. The hard work exists only if there is no interest in what you're doing or no benefit that you can look forward to. There are plenty of benefits to be had from many different types of new challenges in every area of life. When it comes to health and fitness, there are many ways that you can keep yourself striving to stay fit or be even fitter.

Setting higher goals could be choosing to exercise a little longer than you normally do. This may involve working up to a higher level of fitness or it may be just a short-term goal for the week. You could also try learning more about muscle strengthening and the different ways there are to gain better muscle tone. When you start exercises to strengthen your muscles, you might want to set higher weight goals or possibly higher repetition goals. Or as you work up to a higher level of fitness, maybe you can go beyond average and strive for a low body-fat percentage—which would require you to count calories in and calories out. Keep in mind that there are many ways to set new goals and new challenges. The most obvious reason to do so is to keep you focused on the many ways you can test your abilities and your limits so that you never slip back into a life of bad habits and bad health.

☙ ALWAYS LOOK FOR
NEW REASONS TO STAY FIT

There are plenty of other reasons to *stay fit* that go beyond good health (or any of the other reasons you've defined). These reasons will help you stay focused on being healthy and maybe doing some good at the same time. For instance, you can enter a competition—maybe you want to try participating in a charity 5k run or bike ride. There are plenty of charity runs at different times of the year that are of great benefit. There is the popular Race for the Cure that helps raise awareness and money for breast cancer research, put on by the Susan G. Komen foundation. In fact, if you want to find out what charities are available and which causes they support, as well as what events they have, go to http://running.timeoutdoors.com/charities/ and do a search. You can search for a name of a charity or do it based on the cause—children's health, cancers, mental health, and many more. Don't be intimidated by many of these events, because there are plenty of people participating who aren't capable of going the distance without a rest of two (or three or more). It's all about health, awareness, and raising money for a good cause. Just get involved.

You could also plan a vacation that will have new or unfamiliar types of physical activities. Take a vacation that will give you the opportunity to try snow skiing, hiking, waterskiing, and bike riding. How about biking in the mountains? (Not easy going up, but lots of fun coming down!) You don't have to be doing that all the time, but spending a half day doing some sort of interesting physical activity—like walking and sightseeing or going for a long hike (backpacking) to a scenic area—will release your body's endorphins and enkephalins and give you that feeling of euphoria. There are plenty of places to go where you can enjoy a scenic walk and experience some type of history or natural beauty. Mount Rushmore and Old Faithful or a trip to Niagara Falls can be enjoyable and a time to get some exercise and fresh air.

LIMIT FOOD CHOICES

One of the easiest ways to fall back into bad habits is to try new foods that you haven't adequately researched. It's okay to sample new foods, but do yourself a favor and choose those that are located in the produce section of your supermarket *or* a new type of fish or seafood. Stick to those basic foods that consist of fruits, vegetables, lean meats, and fish and you will be fine. You can experiment with healthy preparations of those foods, but my advice is *don't get wrapped up with recipes and new foods.* There will be plenty of times that you will have to eat a variety of meals—holidays, birthdays, special gatherings.

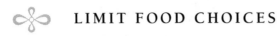 MANAGE YOUR TIME EFFICIENTLY

Now that you've got your healthy habits in place and a new commitment to health in the form of good, nutritious meals, what can you do to make it easier to maintain your fitness level? Another way to be sure you continue on this road is to manage your time efficiently. Even as you try to move up a fitness level, you may find it a bit more difficult to stick to the schedule of exercise each day that you've set for yourself. You may start to feel the limits of what and how much you can do with the time you have. You may be at the point where you know to what degree you feel you want to commit to these ongoing healthy habits.

To improve your level of health, you may have to juggle your schedule in some way and use your time more efficiently. The way to do that is to get more done in less time. For example, make a list of all of your weekly errands and complete them in one afternoon rather than running around here and there every day. You can prepare twice as much when cooking to allow for leftovers. These are just two suggestions, but as you start to value your time more, you will squeeze in what you have to where you can so that your time is more your own. You can also create more time by waking up a little bit earlier.

Ways to Create Time

1. Sleep thirty minutes less (but at least six hours).
2. Work more efficiently—allow only so much time for each task.
3. Prioritize the scheduled tasks from most important to least.
4. Delegate. You don't need to be superhuman—let others do their share.
5. Don't volunteer for everything—stick to your most important causes.

 ## TAKE PREVENTATIVE STEPS TO REMOVE TOXINS

A widely discussed problem that is gaining more and more attention has to do with the health of our colon. As you learned in earlier pages, it has been reported that there are sometimes pounds of waste left in our colon as we approach retirement years. This is apparently due to an accumulation of waste—I'm guessing mainly from poor food choices. Over the past several decades the soil used to grow crops has diminished in quality, the number of less-than-optimal foods has increased in our supermarkets, and fast-food restaurants have flourished. Combine these factors with a diet that involves all three—fewer vitamins and minerals, and more salt and fat—and you have the formula for clogging the colon.

Your colon delivers nutrition to your body and eliminates waste that's unusable or that is finished being used by the body. Picture the food that you eat as having to pass through tiny holes in this tube to get to where it is needed. Some of the substances are passed on (and out) and some are broken down and absorbed through these tiny holes. Over many years, when unhealthy food choices have been made (fatty, oily foods), the tube can become clogged with some of these "leftovers" and even clog some of those tiny holes. Besides making better food choices, you need to "clean out" what is already there with a good colon-cleansing program.

Many experts recommend an annual cleansing, and it is probably a good idea, because the waste that builds up in the colon can be responsible for sickness, disease, improper nutrition, or overall poor health.

Check with your healthcare provider or a nutritionist who is very familiar with maintaining a healthy bowel as to what they would recommend for you.

VISUALIZE A BALANCED LIFE

Losing weight is just one of the reasons that you should be doing this plan. But I don't think you will have a great deal of success if you focus only on the weight you want to lose, or how much you now weigh. It is important to adjust your mindset to one of *living* a healthy lifestyle. Often, we say we want to lose weight but our focus becomes so directed on weight loss that we lose sight of what we need to do each day to reach that goal—water, healthy foods, exercise.

One important way to keep you moving on the road to healthy living is constantly creating a picture in your mind of the type of lifestyle you'd like. In fact, even if you are at the level of health and fitness you are happy with, it's important to reinforce this vision of health so that you don't forget the person *you are*: one who is always practicing what you think—a life filled with health and fitness. When you start visualizing the life you are creating, ask yourself some questions that will help paint that picture.

- What fitness level do you want to realize?
- What job are you doing?
- What activities are you engaging in?
- What is different in the life you have today?
- What are you wearing?
- What types of foods are you eating?
- How do others describe you?
- What exercises do you challenge yourself with?
- What is your energy level?

Think of some of the things that you may be missing out on or that you might be depriving yourself of because of extra weight or because you *think you can't* do because you're not as fit as you *think* you need to be. Have you ever thought

1. "I will do _____ when I lose weight"?
2. "My life will get better after I lose weight"?
3. "I can't do _____ because of my weight"?
4. "That person won't be interested in me because of my weight"?
5. "They won't hire me because of my weight"?
6. "My problems will go away if I lose weight"?
7. "I will be able to eat _____ after I lose the weight"?

There are false beliefs that can be transformed into empowering statements.

- **"If I don't start doing _____ now, I may never lose weight."** If you think you have to wait until you lose weight to go hiking, don't. Start hiking NOW. Or whatever it is, do it now—it will help you lose the weight *and keep it off.*
- **"If I wait in hope that life will get better, things may never improve."** Get busy, improve what you can, and take charge NOW. Your life is in your hands, not anyone else's. Don't wait.
- **"If I think I can't, I'm right. But if I think I can, I'm right."** You may not be able to take the shortest route to the top of a mountain at your current weight, but you can walk around it and go up gradually. You'll eventually reach the summit, so start now because you can!
- **"Anyone not interested in me now is not worthy of consideration later either."** Your weight doesn't need to determine your beauty. Beauty comes from within. Know that you are working to lose weight and that the fat is NOT a personality trait. Stand tall and let yourself shine NOW. The weight will come off when you believe in yourself and will make you healthier. If a person is rude to you now because of your weight, they're not worth considering for a date as you lose weight anyway.
- **"I am capable of doing a good job because I care."** Don't let weight stand in the way of being a valuable asset to any company. You may unleash potential with better health, but that's no different from the many other obstacles that every one of us faces when trying to be, do, and have.

- **"My problems are only problems if I don't take charge to solve them."** You will still have problems when you are thin, they just won't be weight-related health problems. Work toward solving your problems now and you'll be empowered to be healthy in all ways.
- **"I don't need to have just one because that food will never be good for me."** Odds are against your having just one. If you have just one of your *food vice* items, you are more likely to have more—many more! If we could handle moderation of these things that control us, we wouldn't have epidemic obesity rates.

You have let your desires and cravings control you for long enough. Make the right choices for your health and peace of mind.

  ## BUSTING VICES TO HEALTHY CHOICES

There comes a time when you no longer need to look at what not to eat or what not to drink. You will have gone without those unhealthy foods and drinks for enough time so that you shouldn't be thinking about them or even craving them. Your focus should be on choosing healthy foods and drinks instead of replacing those items that were weight killers.

You will get to a point where you won't have diet vices in your life. Sure, there may be areas that you can improve—maybe to help others while helping yourself. Those doughnuts or pastries that are brought to work can be replaced with a fruit tray and some granola. You can make more situations that you come across healthier in order to support the cause. Take a proactive role in providing health all around you as opposed to avoiding and breaking bad or unhealthy habits. Once you have your own weight and health under control, you may find that you can make your life easier while improving the lives around you.

TIME AND EFFORT

Time and effort are two things that are necessary to improve your fitness level. You *can* control the amount of effort you put into making a healthy life for yourself. That effort comes down to not just what you put forth to exercise, but every decision you make that directly or indirectly influences your health in some way. It goes without saying, of course, that the overall plan here is designed to help you make a gradual shift in the direction that ultimately leads to only healthy decisions. I think it is important to reiterate, though, that good health is not a part-time thing. You've probably been kidding yourself more and more over the past twenty years that you can eat right half the time, exercise every so often, live a little bit too free on the weekends, and still be healthy. Well, you can't, and you shouldn't. Progress comes from putting forth the effort each day but also gaining the wisdom to realize that it's only a matter of time before your body will catch up to your actions.

There are many factors about time that seem to be out of your control. The many chemical reactions, including fat mobilization from your body, are just not something that you should realistically think you can change overnight. Like waiting for paint to dry, you don't want to waste time watching and waiting. Time moves at its own pace, and there seem to be many other factors that can alter your perception of time as it goes by (or slows down), but you can "hurry up" the process. This is why it's important to focus on actions, and time will take care of the physical changes.

One woman I worked with, Lisa, just wasn't having any success, and I felt that I was failing her as much as she felt she was failing. Well, I decided to give her an ultimatum: "Drink only water for one week or I'm going to have to discontinue our weekly appointments." She stuck to her guns and drank only water for the week (with the exception of one glass of wine for her sister's birthday). During our next call I told her that she would have to go another week with only water as her beverage, and that I didn't want any excuses. The next week I was not only happy to hear that she had stuck to her commitment, but that she was down 10 pounds (although I'm not a fan of the scale, remember). She went on to lose another 37 pounds over a four-month period. What was holding her up in the beginning was she just didn't think that one or two actions were going to make a difference. She didn't realize that every action takes time to produce a result. It took time for the weight to get there and it was going to take time for it to come off.

❧ HEALTHY THOUGHTS = HEALTHY BODY

It is also important to focus your efforts on moving your mind from where it is to where it needs to be—thinking of all things healthy. Don't be someone who talks about losing weight and chats about it to friends—only to let everyone know that *you know* you need to lose weight—but one who doesn't take action. When you approach losing weight by doing a diet you may not win. When you approach losing weight by changing your mind about what it takes to be healthy, and changing your thoughts from destructive ones to productive, positive, and healthy ones, then you *will win*.

Many health problems are caused by what goes on in our head that we can't measure. Science has shown how negative or destructive thoughts can be damaging to our bodies. In his book *Deadly Emotions* (2003, Thomas Nelson), Dr. Don Colbert describes patients who have been healed through a change of heart by letting go of past painful or negative emotions and moving on toward a peaceful state of mind. Your brain is the control center that sends signals via the nervous system to (ultimately) every cell in the body. Now, imagine that the circuits (your brain and nerves) are shorting out to some degree because of some type of energy interference. That energy interference is your negative thoughts and they ultimately can cause a reduction in your body's ability to function optimally.

Dr. Colbert explains: "The brain regulates the body's immune response and when the regulatory influence of the brain is disrupted, the result may *not* be a lessening of the immune response but an *overstimulation* of it." He goes on to say, "The result is that the body's immune system runs in high gear . . . and fights against even *healthy* cells." This is just one example of the power that less-than-positive emotions can have. Imagine the power of positive emotions.

Positively influencing your emotions on a regular basis—to keep your mind focused on what's good in any situation—is truly the key to having a healthy body. There are too many hurdles to face in life that will wreak havoc on a negative-attitude mind and push you back to square one if you don't possess a positive outlook.

If you're not moving toward healthier and more positive thoughts *on a daily basis,* then you are moving toward unhealthy and negative thoughts. A negative mental attitude can eventually translate into poor health (physical, mental, social, financial, or spiritual). You may get colds or sickness, or a more serious illness may develop. While your negative thoughts don't necessarily make you sick they can get in the way of taking care of yourself, eating right, and exercising.

On the *positive* side, science is just beginning to show some results of the effects of positive thinking. Dr. Herbert Benson, a cardiologist and associate professor of medicine at Harvard, author of ten books, and founder of the Mind/Body Institute in Boston, says, "Mind-body medicine is now scientifically proven." He goes on to say, "When a person can focus on something other than illness, it allows the body to take advantage of our own healing capacity."*

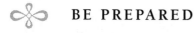 **BE PREPARED**

There are too many places and situations you may find yourself in that present unhealthy varieties or options. Less-than-optimal choices are everywhere you go—you drive by them, walk by them, see them at the checkout counter, and are offered them by coworkers. Being prepared to meet the temptations and distractions is the best way to overcome them.

Prepare to Be Healthy

Carry an attitude of conviction. When you are at work, at home, or out at any social function or get-together, it is bound to happen: You face the temptation of some delicious-looking appetizers, sweets, or other

*As reported in *USA Today*—www.usatoday.com/news/health/2004-10-12-mind-body_x.htm.

tasty calorie-filled foods. What do you do? You carry yourself with an attitude of conviction—a conviction to being healthy and holding firm to your resolve that no food will keep you down, or stand in the way of your reaching your health and fitness goal, *and maintaining that goal.* Your mind can be the one thing that can make or break you—use it to break what's unhealthy that stands in the way. More than what just a little damage one bite will do, the benefit of being strong mentally will build more confidence and conviction, and ultimately you will end up with great shape and health.

Equip yourself with a good defense. The best way to defend against temptations (and let's face it, we're not going to be strong enough to say no *all* of the time), is to come equipped with a defense against those temptations. Having water with you at all times can help—it can suppress your appetite, serves as a substitute for other drinks, and having something in your hand is a great defense. Having an extra, healthy snack with you for those "emergencies" is also recommended. Sugarfree gum is a low-calorie way to keep from having that unhealthy food or beverage.

Know your reasons for choosing health. Of course you want to be healthy and fit, but that is an overall objective for your life. Eating or drinking a *vice* isn't going to spoil a life of good habits and health, but it can. Remember, your fitness level is nothing more than a result of the cumulative decisions you've made over the past few months. You need immediate reasons for saying no and making healthy choices, and that could be because you're going to exercise this afternoon and you don't want to feel sluggish. I think you'd be surprised if you knew that the real reason those few people at work don't participate in company snacks, happy hours, or birthday cakes is because they're *going to the gym later.* It's not easy to get yourself to the gym (or to go exercise) when you feel sluggish from having some high-calorie or high-sugar snack or drink. Think about all the other things you might want to get done today and say no to the unhealthy food or drink in the name of productivity. There's only so much time to get done what you want to get done today.

Reward yourself for making healthy choices. Believe it or not, when you've got that special something planned for the end of the week for having stuck to your commitment to health, you will be more motivated to make the right decisions. Now you've got something else to look forward to that goes beyond what feels like instant gratification and becomes much greater long-term satisfaction and fulfillment. You get to be healthy, have more energy, a better figure—*and a reward!* Maybe you're getting a thirty-minute massage at the end of the week or buying that new CD. This will be the kicker that gives you that extra motivation to make healthy choices.

 ## ARE YOU DIETING?

Finally, if anyone asks if you're *dieting* because of your new decisions to say no, answer, *"I'm doing this great approach to losing weight."* If you want to go further, then say ". . . *and getting healthy and fit."* It will fit in with not telling people you are on a diet, because you're really not. It will keep your answer basic and simple, and you will be promoting the right way to stay on track and live healthily.

 ## TWO SIDES OF HEALTH

Your decisions determine whether you are moving in the direction of better health or not. If you had a piece of pie but ate healthily the rest of the day, you certainly aren't worse off (assuming a normal-size piece) and your actions are on the side of *excellent health,* although the pie alone would not be. Look at the big picture, but take the measure of what you are doing and eating that is having some effect on your overall health. One piece of pie is not going to hurt you, *but* is it going to help? Maybe it will hurt in ways that you might not realize— maybe your energy level dips just enough that you don't feel like exercising later, or at least not at the level you're used to.

At some point in your progress, though, there will come a time when you will go a couple of days or more without an action *against poor health.* (This assumes that you want to improve your level of health and fitness and maintain a higher level.)

The important thing here is not just how to reach a level of optimal health (or a higher level of health and fitness), but understanding how to *avoid poor health.* Most of your actions—either what you do or choose to eat—can be separated into *promotes good health* or *promotes poor health,* with some smaller percentage of things being put into the *neutral* category. Then you'll be able to say no much more easily to those things that won't help you live a life of health.

You will be better off in the long run to eliminate those things that you know either (a) are very tempting to you and can throw you way off track—a diet vice or (b) are just not good anyway, no matter how often you have, do, or eat it. Thinking like this can take the complication out of *dieting* and put you in control. Leave yourself that small window for those special occasions where you will have one piece of pumpkin pie or some wedding cake—but leave it to only those *very* special occasions and you'll be fine.

Secrets to Staying Fit—
Inside and Out

One thing is certain: you will always have some new problem, difficulty, or hurdle to face at some point in your life, big or small. Sometimes these difficulties can lead to setbacks in achieving your health and fitness goals. There are some secrets or tricks that can have your mental and physical health moving to higher levels.

Improving Health & Fitness
Incorporate each tip into your daily life . . .
one at a time.

- Schedule time to relax and recover.
- Set new and challenging goals.
- Focus on new reasons to stay fit.
- Limit your food choices.
- Manage your time efficiently.
- Take preventative steps to remove toxins.
- Visualize a well-balanced, fit, and healthy life.
- Focus more on healthy choices, less on vice busting.
- Continue putting forth a bit of effort and a bit of time.

(continued)
- Keep your thoughts healthy (and your body will be, too).
- Prepare yourself each day to live healthily.
- Proclaim that you've found a healthy approach to losing weight.
- Focus on choices that influence your health positively.
- Life is short so don't wait—*take responsibility now!*

 ## FORGIVENESS

Over the years, I have learned that when it comes to overcoming any difficulties and moving toward goals, we need forgiveness. If you've ever overindulged in unhealthy eating (once or many times) in the past—such as having a chocolate ice-cream fest—and you knew it's not what you should be doing to lose weight and be healthy, then you can't help feeling guilty later. Even if you've gained weight gradually over the years (as is most common) with, for example, a few chocolate-chip cookies each day, you can feel guilty by continuing this habit. By *choosing* to eat those cookies (or whatever it's been over the years—for me, it was ice cream) every day, you're probably accumulating a nice pile of guilt. The pain continues and grows all the while you sabotage (punish) yourself with more poor choices—even though you may be fooling yourself into thinking that it's comforting.

Once you became more aware of the causes of your weight gain, you no doubt experienced a bit of disgust or disappointment with yourself if you then continued to partake of those actions. We've all done it, and chances are good that you may indulge again in something that will make you *feel* bad physically and/or mentally. You can wipe the mental slate clean with forgiveness.

Take the time to sit back and relax, and just for a moment think about and reflect on the past and all those moments that you think were the *cause* of your weight and any painful memories. Then take a deep breath and exhale while letting them all go in the name of forgiveness—because we're all human and we all make mistakes. In fact, mark them down as "learning experiences." You've got to let it go because *it's okay*. Forgiveness allows you to move forward and leave the past behind. If you don't, you may find yourself falling back into that destructive behavior because of your *past* behavior—a vicious cycle. Forgiveness is a very powerful release that will ultimately lead to better mental and physical health.

I think you'd agree that if you want any amount of lasting physical health, you've got to have good mental health. Learn to let go of past mistakes, and when you slip during your healthy lifestyle in the future, the quicker you can confront the situation, learn from it, and forgive yourself, the quicker you can move on and get right back on track. In fact, if you want to add more strength to your mindset, you can adjust your daily affirmations to read

---

 Daily Positive Affirmation

I have unlimited confidence in my abilities and myself. I am thankful for the endless opportunities that each day provides. I forgive myself for any unhealthy actions today, and I welcome optimal health into my life!

 ## PLATEAU BUSTING

The time may come when you've gone a month without dropping any weight. You haven't lost a pound according to the scale (which you're not supposed to be using as a measure of your progress). You've weighed yourself and don't see more than a pound difference from where you were a month or so ago—what do you do? You don't weigh! I can't stress enough that getting on the scale will only lead to frustration. In theory, you could have a very successful month on this program: you could lose 6 pounds of body fat while at the same time building 5 pounds of muscle, your clothes could be one size smaller, but the scale will only show a loss of mere ounces. If you are pound focused you'll be disappointed; however, if you are action focused you will be celebrating that for months you have not had soft drinks, are drinking the water that your body needs, have not eaten fast-food junk, are wearing pants from years ago, *and* are exercising for perhaps the first time in years! That is a success story, regardless of what the scale says.

I teach most clients to view a plateau as a *brief pause*. I've encountered three possibilities that cover most plateaus. The first is that your body needs **time to adjust**. Let's say you may have been losing 8 to 12 pounds a month and now you've lost only 2 pounds. You may just be going through an adjustment period in which your body needs time to catch up.

The second possibility for hitting a plateau is that your diet has not completely attained an **optimum level**. Maybe there is a habit that is slowing you down. Have you reached the point of eating healthily more than 90 percent of the time? Do you have vices that need to be replaced? If you're still moving uphill—meaning building healthy actions, not necessarily getting the weight off—until you've completed the plan and fully established the healthy habits that are outlined, you can't worry about a plateau. On the other hand, if it's six months after you started, then you need to examine the question of how well you're eating. Remember, healthy living and fitness is not a part-time activity—you need to constantly feed yourself with healthy foods.

The final reason you may have hit a plateau—and this holds true for the majority of people who have stuck to a plan for at least a few months—is that you just **need to do more**. More exercise, with more intensity and/or duration. That means make the exercise **harder** for the same amount of time, or make the exercise **longer** by doing the same thing but increasing the time, or do the same exercise but do it **more often**—maybe add another day or two per week. Increasing the difficulty will build more strength; increasing the time you do your exercise will build more stamina.

It's possible that you need to add (or *do more of*) muscle-strengthening exercises. Increasing your muscle tone will help burn more fat while you're *not exercising*. In fact, I have found weight training to be the greatest way to break through almost any health and fitness plateau where an individual already has at least an average diet and a regular schedule of aerobic exercise.

Plateau-Busting Strategies

- Be patient
- Finish this plan
- Check for diet vices
- Add more exercise

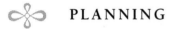 ## PLANNING

A common reason that momentum is lost as you move on with your healthy lifestyle is that the daily written plan or schedule you had starts to slip from view. As you gain more confidence and experience *some* success (weight loss), it's easy to forget about all the things you did to get to there. We all get into a routine—get up at a certain hour, be at work by a certain time, get to the gym by a certain time, eat at a certain time, and go to bed around the same time—almost every day. Having that routine down and those habits formed, you may start to think that you're now in control and you start to leave parts out of the equation. Remember, one of the many things that make you feel "in control" is your written daily plan. Be sure to use a planner or journal. You can see it and remember that you have written down the things you know are necessary to do; the things that hold you accountable to your good health, so don't let them fade from the forefront of your mind.

There are many reasons that having a plan in writing is important to your ongoing improvement and/or maintaining good health and fitness. Let's summarize what the most important reasons are:

Benefits of Having a Written Daily Plan in Your Datebook or Journal

1. Tasks become more important.
2. You become committed to getting them done.
3. You become accountable to good health.
4. You can't "forget" to get them done.

We all have a lot to do each day. I'm sure there are even more things that you would like to do but feel you don't have the time for. Having a written plan helps you to budget your time and see where there are openings for taking on new actions. You can start that new hobby, education, or service that you've always wanted to do when you can see where it will fit into your schedule. You will also be able to see what you might be doing that isn't as important as you once thought, so you can make room for that other something that has been on your mind for months (or years).

Here's what I think happens to many of us as we age. We get busy doing quite a few things from work, to household chores, children's activities, and so on. We often think about many other things and engage in conversation with friends or family about these things. Over the years many new and different creative ideas and thoughts pop into our minds. If we don't write down those ideas and pursue them, at some point our minds won't feel like giving us any more ideas because they never *get used*. Be it a new degree, a new craft, a new activity, service, charity, volunteer work, campaign, or whatever—you've got to reinforce your mind that these things are worth consideration. They are worth considering because *you thought of it*! The way to be sure you consider your new ideas is to *write them down when you think of 'em*. Make them part of your ongoing plan that involves new and stimulating thoughts—you never know where any of those thoughts might lead.

⚜ HYGIENE

Believe it or not, improved hygiene is an excellent way to maintain your momentum toward optimal health. Good hygiene is also important to *maintain* optimal health and is a great way to reinforce your commitment to being healthy.

There are many ways that you can improve your hygiene that you might not have thought of. For example, brushing your teeth after *every* meal and *every* snack, and using a good breath rinse afterward, could discourage you from eating snacks that are easy to hide and eat throughout the day.

Improve the quality of the air you breathe by using an air purifier.

According to the Environmental Protection Agency (EPA),* "The short-term [health effects from indoor air pollutants] can cause irritation of the eyes, nose, and throat, headaches, dizziness, and fatigue. Such immediate effects are usually short-term and treatable. Symptoms of some diseases, including asthma, hypersensitivity pneumonitis, and humidifier fever, may also show up after exposure to some indoor air pollutants." An air purifier that is a "highly efficient collector of pollutants and has a high air-circulation rate" is the ideal type to have, according to the EPA. Make your home a clean place to live *and breathe*!

Taking the time to keep your kitchen and the rest of your home, your clothes, your car, where you work (and your body) clean and neat will reinforce your commitment to health throughout your life. If you've taken the time to organize and clean all of the places that you are and will be, then you certainly won't want to spoil your self-image by putting something "dirty" (unhealthy) in your body.

Wash your hands more often. Living on a high level of health and fitness requires actions that are always supporting good health, and hand washing is one of them. According to the Centers for Disease Control (CDC), "The most important thing you can do to keep from getting sick is washing your hands."†

Let it be your attitude to continue to strive for all things healthy. It's only in this way that you can be assured of never having a weight problem again.

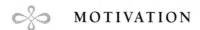   **MOTIVATION**

If you've accomplished everything you set out to accomplish in your life, your goals were too small. If you can check off each of your goals because you feel you reached them—be they health related, job related, or in any other area of your life—you may feel a complete lack of motivation to continue doing more and greater things. There is always something more that you can do. If you don't think so, then there is *always* someone else you can help.

*From www.epa.gov/iaq/pubs/insidest.html
†From the CDC's Web site: www.cdc.gov/ncidod/op/handwashing.htm

Motivation is not willpower, it isn't something you are born with, and it isn't something that you get from somewhere else. Focusing on only losing weight can be very unmotivating, consuming you with an attitude of "don't do this" and "don't do that" and "must avoid this" and "can't eat that." Motivation comes from realizing what you're missing out on that you could be putting your focus and attention toward. Motivation is choosing to "see" what you did not see before—it's a cause-and-effect relationship. You realize the effect that is possible from taking action and becoming healthier.

Again, here are some of the typical reasons that people have for wanting to lose weight:

- To have more energy
- To feel attractive
- To be sexy again
- To think more clearly
- To find a life partner
- To wear cute clothes
- To live longer
- To achieve more goals
- To feel more confident
- To be the person you know you can be

It's also important to look beyond those reasons, because you may just find that there are many more possibilities when you reach a higher level of health and fitness. You have endless potential.

HANDLING COMMON STUMBLES

You are bound to have struggles, stumbles, or slip-ups. We all do. You have to decide that what you're striving for is **good** in all senses of the word—it helps your health inside and out and the effects on others will be positive (directly or indirectly).

You will find that the more effort you put toward your health, the more you will learn. And the more you learn and do, the more opportunity you have to "fail" or achieve a different or unwanted result. The knowledge and the experience that you will gain will overshadow any disappointment. Not only that, but remember how you should judge your life: how well you handle adversity. If you handle disappointments, unwanted results, unusual effects, or difficulties with anger, resentment, hostility, or extreme sadness—all for any length of time—you will ultimately conclude that life is nothing but a disappointment, which it's not. Remember that **everyone** has small *and* big problems to deal with—it all comes down to how you choose to handle them.

Handling a Stumble

1. Don't make a mountain out of a molehill—it happens.
2. Decrease the length of time you're down—so you're not out.
3. Work on decreasing the frequency with which they happen.
4. Decide to handle adversity with conviction and a positive attitude.
5. Put a smile on your face and keep going.

 ## FINAL THOUGHTS

Dear friend,

I hope you have enjoyed this journey and will continue on so that you can live all of your dreams. Remember that weight loss is just the by-product of healthy choices and positive actions, and that all the other positive benefits of losing weight will be the motivators behind those healthy and positive actions. Those choices you make will ultimately decide whether you will get to a healthy weight and continue to remain at a healthy weight. Make the decision to choose a healthy lifestyle.

A healthy lifestyle is not a destination—it is a journey!

Make it your life's pursuit to make every area of your life healthy—your mind, your body, your spirit, your relationships, your job, your hobbies, and so on. The thought of how much potential every one of us has is really exciting—especially if you consider all the claims that we are using less than 20 percent of our brain (or something close). Tap into some of that potential and see where it could lead you.

Ultimately, you have to take full responsibility for you actions, your results, and your life! It is only then that you can achieve the results that you desire.

I wish you the best and ask that you visit me on my Web site with comments, questions, **and your success story!** I'd love to hear from you. Go to www.vicebusting.com.

Yours in health,

Julia

Carpe Diet!

Afterword

As an oncologist who has been practicing for over twenty years, I see the end result of poor nutrition and lifestyle choices. Diseases that were once seen only in older adults are now becoming commonplace in children and young people. Obesity, hypertension, diabetes, and cancer are epidemic. New diseases such as fibromyalgia and chronic fatigue syndrome have been described to encompass symptoms that are increasingly afflicting our modern society. We have a generation of children with behavioral problems and learning disabilities and adults with early onset dementia and Alzheimer's. What in the world is happening? America has the most sophisticated medical care in the world, but we are far from healthy.

Julia Havey is one of those people who gets it: Obesity is not just a cosmetic problem; obesity kills.

My specialty is breast cancer. Twenty-five years ago, when I first started my career in medicine, breast cancer affected older women. My practice now includes a large percentage of women who are in their twenties, thirties, and forties—and the incidence rises every year!

Being overweight increases the risk of breast cancer. And among those who already have the disease, obese women have a higher risk of recurrence and a poorer survival rate. Obesity also increases the risk of other major diseases, including heart disease, stroke, and diabetes. And then there are obesity-related symptoms that occur prior to being labeled with a diagnosis, such as fatigue, joint pain, back problems, insomnia, and depression. The costs related to obesity are staggering.

Unfortunately, nutrition and healthy eating remain a mystery to most families. Julia Havey helps to solve that mystery. I became a nutritionist out of necessity: My patients and their families kept asking me questions about the foods that they should be eating and the supplements that they should take. Like most mainstream physicians, I had few answers, as nutrition and prevention of disease are not a large part of most medical school curricula. When my own debilitating health problems started in my midforties (chronic fatigue, daily low back pain, and joint pain), I made a commitment to myself and to my patients to become educated in the relationship between diet and disease. I now attend medical conferences on alternative and preventative medicine for my continuing education credits, and I devour articles and books on nutrition and health.

The truth is that the vast majority of people can attain ideal health, and the sooner one begins, the better. Julia Havey puts the responsibility where it belongs—on the individual. Obesity and its dire consequences can be reversed and prevented. We have choices. I chose to reverse my own poor health, and I now empower others to do the same through education, support, and love.

I am especially drawn to the young women in my practice with children yet to raise, as I have witnessed far too many times how poor health can destroy families. The information that I have learned has revitalized my practice, and—like Julia Havey—I share my knowledge and passion with others. My health lectures locally and around the country have been attended by thousands of people who are hungry for the truth. The image of the doctor with one hand on the door and the other hand on the prescription pad is no longer acceptable! We have a responsibility to families and to the world at large to reverse the dangerous downward spiral of poor health. Like Julia, I want to be remembered as someone who is making a difference.

I am commonly asked about nutritional supplements. Although supplements are never a substitute for food, the reality is that 90 percent of Americans do not consume the nine to thirteen daily servings of fruits and vegetables recommended by the American Cancer Society and American Heart Association for good health. Even if we did eat perfectly every day, today's fruits and vegetables too often lack the nutrition that they had decades ago. Processed foods have little nutritional value and cooking can deplete food of its nutrients. For example, microwaving can destroy up to 90 percent of the nutrients in vegetables.

Bridging the nutritional gaps that we all have is crucial to our good health. The only nutritional product that I have ever taken or given to my children is Juice Plus+®.

As a physician, the only thing that I have at the end of the day is my reputation, so I have made a rule of not endorsing any of the hundreds of nutritional supplements that various companies have bombarded me with over the years. Juice Plus+® is the exception to this rule, because there is a growing body of independent clinical research on the product that has been published or is under way in a variety of populations worldwide. Research published to date in peer-reviewed medical journals shows that Juice Plus+® is bioavailable, raises antioxidant levels, lowers lipid peroxides (free radicals) and homocysteine, enhances immune function, protects DNA integrity, and helps maintain normal blood flow. No prescription drug or vitamin or mineral supplement can do all that! Because it is whole-food based, Juice Plus+® provides thousands of phytonutrients (including vitamins and minerals) that our bodies need.

I hope that Julia's story will empower and motivate you to learn more about your health and nutrition. Turn off the television, take an honest look at your diet and lifestyle choices, and begin immediately to take the steps to change your health, your future, and that of your family.

Life is not a dress rehearsal. Don't wait until you receive your wake-up call; by then it may be too late!

Delia M. Garcia, M.D., F.A.C.R.,
Radiation Oncology,
St. Louis, Missouri

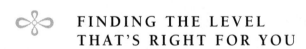 *Appendix I*

Levels of Health and Fitness

FINDING THE LEVEL
THAT'S RIGHT FOR YOU

When it comes to exercise, we are faced with a situation very much like that of trying to lose weight: If we are to be successful, we need the **right approach.** The wrong approach involves too much too fast that we can't possibly live with for the rest of our life. When two people buy the same piece of exercise equipment but have completely different fitness levels—one very fit and one who has done very little exercise—the one with little experience will most likely quickly lose interest in the equipment after a short time.

You need to start exercising at a level that is suitable for your level of health and fitness. Once you've found your level, you need to first develop the habit, then worry about increasing the frequency, duration, and intensity of your exercise.

The levels of health and fitness will give you an idea of where to start, based on your overall health and fitness. You can make the determination of your level based on the greatest number of criteria that describe you.

Each level will also provide a better understanding and expectation of the goals you want to reach—how much effort and how much time it will take to reach the next level when implementing this plan.

A few variables factor into each level. The first variable is genetics. Don't let your genetics become an excuse as to why you can't lose weight and get fit.

A second variable is the difference between men and women. This is also accounted for to some degree with the range of time needed to move to the next level. But it doesn't account for the fact that men have a higher metabolism than women.

The third variable is what happens with age. When you age your metabolism will slow down and your hormone levels will be the lowest they've been in years (or your entire life).

While reading through each of the following pages, make two determinations:

1. **What is my current level of health and fitness?**
2. **What level of health and fitness would I like to reach?**

Once you can identify *your* level, you know where to start. And once you choose what level you'd like to be at (the one you will be *visualizing* each day), you'll start to get an idea of the time it takes and how much effort you'll need to get there *and* stay there.

There is a difference in being at a healthy weight and being physically fit. The levels of health and fitness are defined to include both. I think you'll agree that by sticking to some simple and basic fundamentals of good health, success is more possible and life is much easier.

Once you start making progress and you begin to reach a higher level, you can start deciding how detailed you want to be about burning a particular number of calories, measuring your basal metabolic rate (BMR)—in short, how much you want to qualify your exercise.

You will notice that each level also has an estimated range of pounds overweight. This is a guideline only. While they represent a good estimate, don't reject the level solely on the basis of this.

Keep in mind that we're all built with varying degrees of power, size, durability, and efficiency—based on our genetics, gender, age, and so on. That doesn't mean we can't be healthy at any level, but not all of the criteria listed for a particular level may apply to us.

Fitness Factors for Each Level:

1. **Degree of physical activity**
2. **Physical endurance/capability**
3. **Pounds of weight loss needed**
4. **Knowledge of health and fitness**
5. **Awareness of health and fitness**
6. **Daily plan or schedule present**
7. **Healthy choices, including meals**
8. **Degree of positive or negative attitude**
9. **Frequency of being ill or sick**
10. **Overall commitment to health**

Please keep in mind that these are guidelines and that there are exceptions and variations. The levels are discussed in the order of beginner level to the highest level of fitness.

Health and Fitness—Beginner, Level I

Qualities of Health and Fitness Level I

Check the box that applies if you are on this level

- ☐ 1. You don't exercise, don't like it, don't want to do it, are fearful of it
- ☐ 2. You have no energy, no endurance—struggle to complete almost any physical task
- ☐ 3. You desire to lose 100 pounds or more
- ☐ 4. Your knowledge of health is limited
- ☐ 5. You are not even aware of how many decisions/thoughts contribute to poor health
- ☐ 6. You have no plan—you're focused on getting the normal few things done as usual
- ☐ 7. You make few, if any, healthy choices—maybe leaving it up to the doctors
- ☐ 8. You feel distraught and hopeless, even fearful
- ☐ 9. For you sickness is a way of life—with or without noticeable symptoms

❑ 10. You likely have never known how to make a commitment to
good health

Some of the qualities that you see listed may not be agreeable to
you, but plenty of improvements can be made at this level that you may
not even be aware of. Maybe you have made some poor health and diet
choices, but you can turn things around. I did. You have to start by accepting the possibility of a life full of health and fitness. Then you have
to accept the probability for a needed mental boost. So pick yourself up
by your bootstraps and let's get going—**one simple step at a time!**

Exercise: **Frequency**: 3 days per week; **Time**: 5–20 minutes; **Intensity**:
easiest; **Suggested Cardio**: walking; **Muscle-strengthening**: none until week 6, then light weights, 20 minutes twice per week. **Summary**:
The biggest key is to get in the habit of doing what you know you can
and stick to at least 3 days per week, and walking is usually the easiest
to perform. If knees and/or other joints are a problem, try using a stationary bike. The goal is to get moving more often and strive to do it for
4 days per week. And be sure to check with your doctor before starting
this, or any, exercise program. The key at this point is to get your body
moving and create the habit of exercise.
Here is a rundown of the basic forms of exercise. These are really
all that you need to get started on the path to fitness. As you progress,
increase intensity, frequency, and/or duration.

SUMMARY OF *BASIC* EXERCISES

Cardio	*Muscle Strengthening*
Easiest—5–20 minutes	**Easiest**
*Slow walking—level surface	3-lb. dumbbells used for overhead
Slow walking on a treadmill (no incline)	lifting, arm curling, deep knee bends with no weight (only basic move-
Slow pace stationary bicycling, no resistance	ments); No more than 12 repetitions for each movement done 3 times per
preferred	week

Cardio	*Muscle Strengthening*
Mild to Easy—(20 minutes) Medium-speed walking (no incline) Medium pace on a treadmill (no incline) Med. speed, low resistance stationary bike Slow-paced swimming with regular 1-min. rests	**Mild to Easy** 5-lb. dumbbells used; 15 repetitions: arm curls, overhead presses, deep knee bends with no weight (only basic movements); 12–15 repetitions for each movement, done 3 times per week
Mild—(20–30 minutes) Medium-speed walking (some minor hills) Medium pace treadmill (slight incline) Medium pace elliptical machine, low resistance Medium pace stationary bike, low resistance Medium pace bicycling, some hills Slow pace swimming with regular 1-min. rests Medium pace rowing, low resistance Low intensity, mild pace aerobic class Beginner kickboxing or other cardio class	**Mild** 10–20-lb. dumbbells; 15 repetitions: arm curls, overhead presses, squatting while holding a broomstick or straight bar behind the neck that is < 10 lbs. **OR** consider starting an easy-circuit training program at a gym; **OR** using an all-in-one home exercise machine—with either, start with 4 simple exercises, low weight, 2 sets with 15 repetitions each set, performed 3 times per week
Moderate—(30–45 minutes) Fast pace walking (some good hills) Fast pace treadmill (medium incline) Fast pace elliptical machine, med. resistance Fast pace stationary bike, medium resistance Fast pace bicycling, some difficult hills Med. pace swimming with regular 45-sec. rests Fast pace rowing, medium resistance	**Moderate** Complete muscle-strengthening exercises: 5 exercises minimum (1 of each)—chest, back, legs, biceps, triceps, shoulders, and abs; 3 sets using medium (level of difficulty) weight with 15 repetitions each set, performed 3 times per week. At this point a gym membership is practically a must-have. The environment and variety of machines will keep you committed to moving up the fitness scale.

Cardio	*Muscle Strengthening*
Medium intensity, medium pace aerobic class Mid-level kickboxing or other cardio class	

High—(45 minutes or more)
Fast pace walking—difficult hills
Fast pace treadmill—med. to hard incline
Fast pace elliptical—med. to hard resistance
Fast pace stationary bike—difficult resistance
Fast pace bicycling—difficult hills
Med. pace swimming—regular 30-second rests
Fast pace rowing—med. to difficult resistance
High intensity, medium pace aerobic class
High-level kickboxing or other cardio class
	High
	Muscle-strengthening routine—half of the muscles on one day, half on the other, with 1 or 2 days off, then repeating those 2 days;
	Ex: Day 1—chest, back, shoulders, abs
	    Day 2—legs, triceps, biceps, abs
	    Day 3 (and 4) off
	    Day 4 (or 5)—Repeat Day 1
	    Day 5 (or 6)—Repeat Day 2
	    Day 6 (or 7)—off

Highest—(1 hour or more)	**Highest**

Time needed to reach Level II: approximately 4 weeks to 3 months

When you have done level I for *at least* four weeks and feel that you are ready for more, go on to Beginner, Level II.

Health and Fitness—Beginner, Level II

Qualities of Health and Fitness Level II

When you are on this level

❏ 1. You don't exercise, haven't done much if any in the past, don't like it

❑ 2. You have little energy and little endurance—struggle to get through each day

❑ 3. You desire to lose 75–100 pounds—maybe put faith in diets for years

❑ 4. You have not much knowledge of healthy living

❑ 5. You are not considering the consequences of any choices as being healthy or not

❑ 6. You have no plan, little hope; you desire to change, but don't know where to begin

❑ 7. You are making poor food and beverage choices; not many healthy choices

❑ 8. Your attitude is chronically poor or negative—maybe not noticeably

❑ 9. You are always taking some form of medicine for something—you're sick way too often

❑ 10. You are concerned about your health but lack motivation—you feel too overwhelmed

If you feel that you can most closely identify with this level of health and fitness, it's time to get moving. You may not like exercise and you might even fear doing it because you feel apprehensive of people watching. You're not alone if you feel this way. Exercise is probably one of the biggest hurdles that you've faced in the past. Hopefully, the simple changes that come before exercise will provide enough of a benefit to get you believing that good health and a better life is truly within your grasp.

Exercise: **Frequency**: 3 days per week; **Time**: 20 minutes; **Intensity**: low or easier; **Suggested Cardio:** walking, treadmill, stationary bike; **Muscle strengthening:** none until Week 6, then light weights, 20 minutes twice per week. **Summary:** Work on getting comfortable doing some form of cardio at least 3 days per week and work up to 4 days per week for 30 minutes; 2 weeks after that point, start some easy muscle-strengthening exercises—small dumbbells that can be used at home doing some basic movements 3 times per week.
Time needed to reach Intermediate Levels: 4 weeks to 3 months before being ready to move on
Before progressing make sure that the Beginner Levels I and II feel comfortable and perhaps even a bit easy.

Health and Fitness—Intermediate, Level III

Qualities of Health and Fitness Level III

When you are on this level

- ❑ 1. You don't exercise, maybe have in the past; not much physical activity
- ❑ 2. You feel sluggish throughout the day—may be consuming too much caffeine
- ❑ 3. You desire to lose 50–75 pounds—you are frustrated and anxious about it
- ❑ 4. You lack knowledge of health—not applying what you do know
- ❑ 5. You are unaware of how some of your choices are harming your health
- ❑ 6. You feel that you have more potential than you show—desire change
- ❑ 7. You eat fruits and vegetables once in a while—maybe to mask the bad foods
- ❑ 8. You show a decent attitude but may be "hurting" inside and negative
- ❑ 9. You take medicines too frequently for some type of sickness
- ❑ 10. You feel overwhelmed and unable to focus on getting healthy

Don't be discouraged if you identify with this level—you're doing something about it. One thing I want to point out that needs a good tune-up: your attitude. As we've discussed, a positive attitude can go a long way toward getting you started and keeping you going in your quest for better health and fitness. A bad attitude—negative, defeatist, or any mood that gets in the way of your achieving your goals—needs to be turned around.

The point here is that at this level you need to focus your thoughts and attitude right now so you can start moving in the right direction and believing that you're capable of more—and what you're capable of is almost *always more than you think.*

Exercise: **Frequency**: 3 days per week; **Time**: 20 minutes; **Intensity**: low to medium; **Suggested Cardio**: walking, treadmill, stationary bike,

swimming; **Muscle strengthening:** machines only 2 days a week 4–6 weeks, working up to 3 days a week; 3 sets per muscle group, 12 repetitions per set. **Summary:** Work on consistency and increasing the cardio to 4 days, then increasing the minutes to 30; start with light weight on the machines.
Time needed to reach Intermediate, Level IV: 4 weeks to 3 months

Health and Fitness—Intermediate, Level IV

Qualities of Health and Fitness Level IV

When you are on this level

- ❑ 1. You are familiar with some exercises but don't get much physical activity
- ❑ 2. You have an average level of endurance—get tired on and off during the day
- ❑ 3. You desire to lose 25–50 pounds—you are worried often about it
- ❑ 4. You have some knowledge of health—nutrition, much of it conflicting
- ❑ 5. You are not as aware of all the causes of the extra weight (poor choices)
- ❑ 6. You are not worried about goals; you live by a daily routine or are in a rut
- ❑ 7. You are not getting enough fruits, vegetables, or lean meats
- ❑ 8. You have a low energy level, hence a less-than-positive attitude
- ❑ 9. You get sick too often and would like to feel healthier more often
- ❑ 10. Your life lacks balance—too little physical activity, too many calories

A large percentage of the population find themselves at this level: 25 pounds or more overweight with not quite the energy level and endurance that's possible. You may not *believe* that you can have more energy and more endurance, but you will be surprised. I think most people just chalk up their low energy and endurance to stress and age—both of which are legitimate reasons for not having the energy of an 18-year-old.

But we're talking about *what's possible for you* as a healthy and fit individual. And it doesn't matter what your age *or stress level,* your health will most likely be compromised if you identify most with this level.

Exercise: **Frequency:** 3 days per week; **Time:** 30 minutes; **Intensity:** low to medium; **Suggested Cardio:** (1) walking, elliptical, treadmill, stationary bike, swimming; (2) dancing, kickboxing, step-aerobics; **Muscle strengthening:** machines only 2 days a week for 3 weeks, working up to 3 days a week; 3 sets per muscle group. **Summary:** Work on consistency and getting to 6 days per week (3 for each).
    Time needed to reach Level V: 4 weeks to 3 months

Health and Fitness—Intermediate, Level V

Qualities of Health and Fitness Level V

When you are on this level

    ❑ 1. You are good at getting regular exercise but sometimes go a few days without
    ❑ 2. You have decent muscle tone and endurance but only when consistently exercising
    ❑ 3. You desire to lose up to 25 pounds; you're not too worried about it—expect to get to it
    ❑ 4. You have a good knowledge of health and fitness; you're not as good at applying it
    ❑ 5. You have a reasonable awareness of what you're eating but are not overly concerned
    ❑ 6. You have a daily routine of habits—not a plan; you schedule things when needed
    ❑ 7. You make healthy choices often enough to keep from gaining more than a few pounds
    ❑ 8. You have a pretty good attitude but you fall well short of your capabilities
    ❑ 9. You have health problems regularly because of your incomplete diet and exercise control
    ❑ 10. You lead a well-balanced life but believe you are capable of better health and fitness

You may be in very good physical condition but you still want to lose another 5 pounds or so. You might have to decide at this point whether it's time to increase your efforts that will put you on the next level. Or you may have closer to 20 or 25 pounds that you *need* to lose—weight that may be hindering your energy, your productivity, and even your health. The biggest problem you may have on this level is the time you can devote to getting enough exercise. You may not have a problem with consuming too many calories, but you're consuming the wrong kind of calories—an occasional gourmet coffee drink, a healthy lunch, maybe, an afternoon sweet, and a healthy dinner.

Exercise: **Frequency:** 3 days per week; **Time:** 40 minutes; **Intensity:** medium to high; **Suggested Cardio:** walking/jogging, stair-stepper, elliptical, treadmill, kickboxing, aerobic classes, or spinning; **Muscle strengthening:** 3 days a week; 3 sets per muscle group. **Summary:** Work up to 40 minutes for cardio and 3 days per week for muscle strengthening.

Time needed to reach Advanced, Level VI: an additional 3 months

Health and Fitness—Advanced, Level VI

Qualities of Health and Fitness Level VI

When you are on this level

❑ 1. You are involved with some sort of exercise almost daily (6 of 7 days)
❑ 2. You are very conditioned with a high endurance level
❑ 3. You have no need to lose weight—you're at or very near an "outstanding" figure
❑ 4. You have and apply adequate knowledge of nutrition and supplementation
❑ 5. You have an excellent diet with awareness of fat/carb/protein content
❑ 6. You have an exercise schedule; consistently plan each day
❑ 7. You most often put healthy choices first over anything else
❑ 8. You have a positive attitude and are an example of good health and fitness

❏ 9. You have infrequent health problems—rarely a cold or flu
❏ 10. You have a great commitment to health; your vacations are used for being active

On this level you have a high degree of dedication to exercise and diet. The difference between this level and the top level is that your lifestyle is a little bit more balanced. A high priority is placed on health and fitness, but it's not *everything*.

Exercise: **Frequency:** 3 days per week; **Time:** 50 minutes; **Intensity:** upper medium to high; **Suggested Cardio:** jogging, cycling, swimming, elliptical, treadmill, stair-stepper, kickboxing, body pump, spinning, or other similar cardio exercises; **Muscle strengthening:** 4 days per week, dividing muscles into two groups—legs, back, and bicep muscles 1 day; chest, shoulders, and triceps muscles another day; ab muscles every day. **Summary:** You decide where to go from here!

Time needed to reach Advanced, Level VII: at least 6 months after arriving at Level V—you can healthfully stay at Level VI for the rest of your life. Level VII is intense and only for those who are very serious about fitness and appearance.

Health and Fitness—Advanced, Level VII

Exercise time per day: 1½ hours or more

Qualities of Health and Fitness Level VII

When you are on this level

❏ 1. You are involved with some sort of physical sport almost daily (min. 6 days)
❏ 2. You are conditioned for high-energy and/or high-endurance competition
❏ 3. You are not concerned about weight; your only concern is staying or getting more fit
❏ 4. You have a vast knowledge of nutrition and supplementation
❏ 5. You are aware of caloric expenditures and caloric intake each day

❑ 6. You have a strict workout/exercise schedule; you live by a daily plan

❑ 7. You choose healthy meals and activities that don't intrude on fitness

❑ 8. You have a positive attitude; you are an example of dedication to fitness

❑ 9. You are rarely sick or have any symptoms of cold or flu; if any, you heal quickly

❑ 10. You have the highest commitment to health; you don't take vacations from health

You are at the highest level of health and fitness. It's a level that is not easy to achieve *or maintain*. For most people, this level may be achieved through pursuit of some fitness goal that requires constant conditioning, like competitive sports or strenuous outdoor activities—rock climbing, marathons, and so on.

Exercises: high-endurance activities; 1 hour of cardio (running, cycling, swimming, elliptical, stair-stepper, treadmill, or similar) and 1 hour of weight-training, usually split into different muscle groups for different days—3 or more days per week; other physical activities are included for another 1 hour or more minimum

Appendix II

Quick and Healthy Recipes

 MORNING FUEL

I can't encourage you enough to find a few basic core meals that are nutritious, fit your lifestyle, and provide your body with proper fuel, and to eat those most often. Spending all day thinking about what to eat, when to eat, and how to make it tends to give food an inordinate amount of importance in your life. Food is fuel—nothing more and nothing less.

Whole Wheat Pancakes
(Serves 4, makes about 8 pancakes)

> 1 cup plus 2 tablespoons whole wheat flour
> 1 tablespoon brown sugar
> 1½ teaspoons baking powder
> pinch of salt
> 2 tablespoons applesauce
> 1 cup plus 2 tablespoons water

Sift all dry ingredients together. Add the applesauce and water and mix until the batter drips from spoon but is not runny. Heat a frying pan and spray it with low-fat cooking spray (Pam). Spoon about ¼ cup of batter into the pan and let it cook until small bubbles form in the center. Flip. Keep the cooked pancakes warm in a preheated oven and cover with a paper towel to keep the moisture in. Serve with a low-fat butter substitute and low-fat maple syrup.

Variation: For a special treat, make the batter with either ½ cup sunflower seeds or ½ cup blueberries.

German Apple-Potato Pancakes
(Serves 4)

> 1¼ cups unpeeled apples, finely chopped
> 1 cup peeled potatoes, grated
> ½ cup applesauce
> ½ cup all-purpose flour
> 2 egg whites
> 1 teaspoon salt

Preheat oven to 475°F. Spray a cookie sheet with nonstick cooking spray.

In a medium bowl, combine all ingredients. Spray a large nonstick skillet with nonstick cooking spray and heat over medium heat until hot. Drop rounded tablespoons of batter 2 inches apart into the skillet. Cook 2 to 3 minutes on each side or until lightly browned. Place pancakes on the prepared cookie sheet. Bake 10 to 15 minutes or until crisp. Serve with additional applesauce or apple slices.

Lemon Pancakes
(Serves 4, makes 8 pancakes—2 per serving)

> 1 egg or egg substitute
> ½ cup lemon fat-free yogurt
> ½ cup skim milk

2 tablespoons oil
1 tablespoon sugar
½ teaspoon nutmeg
1 cup all-purpose flour
1 teaspoon baking powder
½ teaspoon baking soda

In a bowl beat the egg and mix in the yogurt, milk, and oil. Stir in the sugar and nutmeg. In a separate bowl combine the flour, baking powder, and baking soda. Add the flour mixture to the liquid and mix. The batter will be thick. Grease a griddle and pour in ¼ cup batter. Cook the pancakes until they bubble, then turn them. Serve with warm maple syrup.

Wheat and Flax Pancakes
(Serves 8, makes 8 large pancakes)

⅓ cup flaxseed, finely ground
1 cup whole wheat flour
1 cup brown rice flour
⅓ cup toasted wheat germ
⅓ cup powdered milk
1½ cups water
1 tablespoon maple sugar or light brown sugar
2½ teaspoons baking powder
½ teaspoon salt

In large bowl whisk together the ground flaxseed, whole wheat flour, brown rice flour, wheat germ, powdered milk, water, sugar, baking powder, and salt. Refrigerate until ready to use. Lightly grease griddle and pour ¼ cup of batter. Cook pancakes until bubbly, flip, cook till lightly done. Serve with light maple syrup.

Variation: Put some sliced banana on top after batter has been poured into pan.

Pumpkin Pie Pancakes
(Serves 4)

1 large egg
½ cup pumpkin puree
1 tablespoon butter, softened
½ teaspoon vanilla extract
2 tablespoons sour cream
¾ cup flour
⅓ cup flaxseed, finely ground
⅓ cup whey protein powder
2 packets Splenda
½ teaspoon cinnamon
¼ teaspoon ginger
¼ teaspoon ground cloves
¼ teaspoon ground allspice
¼ teaspoon baking powder
¼ teaspoon baking soda

In a medium bowl lightly beat the egg. Blend in the pumpkin, butter, vanilla, and sour cream. In a separate bowl sift together all dry ingredients. Combine wet and dry ingredients. Mix well. On a lightly greased skillet, dollop out about ⅓ cup of batter to make each pancake. Cook until done.

Onion and Tomato Scramble
(Serves 1)

½ cup green onions, sliced
4 small cherry tomatoes
3 egg whites
Pinch of fresh basil, chopped
Pinch of fresh parsley, chopped

Put sliced onion in an oiled pan. Cook on medium heat until they start to change color, about 4 minutes. Meanwhile, slice and dice the tomatoes, discarding the juice, and add it to the pan with the onions. Cook for about 2 minutes. Beat the egg whites and pour them into the pan.

Add the chopped basil and cook, stirring constantly, until ready. Garnish with parsley.

Easy Mexican Eggs
(Serves 1)

> 3 egg whites
> 1 egg yolk
> 1 tablespoon salsa (Paul Newman's—helps a good cause)
> Finely diced jalapeños to taste

Mix all ingredients together in a bowl. Pour into a Pam-sprayed pan and heat at medium-low. Cook slowly until done to your liking.

Variation: Sprinkle on a bit of grated jalapeño jack cheese to taste.

Eggsplant Benedict
(Serves 4)

> ½ cup fresh basil leaves
> 1 teaspoon minced garlic
> 2 tablespoons pine nuts
> Salt and pepper to taste
> ½ cup olive oil
> ¼ cup grated Parmesan
> 1 tablespoon olive oil for brushing
> Four ½-inch-thick tomato slices
> Four ½-inch-thick eggplant slices
> 2 English muffins, halved
> 4 eggs

In a food processor mix the basil, garlic, pine nuts, salt, and pepper until well combined. Add ¼ cup of the oil and puree. Add the remaining oil and the cheese and mix until blended. Brush tomato and eggplant slices with oil and roast in a preheated 375°F oven for 5 minutes, turning once. Lightly brush the muffins with pesto (the basil mixture) and toast under the broiler. Poach the eggs.

To assemble, put a muffin on a plate and stack the tomato and eggplant on each serving. Carefully place an egg on top and drizzle with pesto.

Popeye's Pie
(Serves 4)

> 1 package (10 ounces) frozen chopped spinach, thawed and well
>   drained
> ½ cup shredded low-sodium Swiss cheese, about 2 ounces
> ¼ cup chopped onion
> ½ cup Cream of Rice cereal, uncooked
> 1½ teaspoons baking powder
> 1½ cups fat-free milk
> ¾ cup Egg Beaters
> 2 tablespoons margarine or butter, melted

Mix the spinach, cheese, and onion in the bottom of greased 9-inch pie plate and set aside. Blend the cereal and baking powder in medium bowl. Stir in the milk, egg product, and margarine. Pour over the spinach mixture. Bake at 400°F for 30 minutes or until puffed and golden. Cut into wedges to serve; garnish as desired.

Crepes
(Serves 5)

> 1 cup low-fat milk
> 1 large egg plus 1 egg white
> ¾ cup whole wheat flour
> 1 tablespoon sugar (optional)

In a blender or food processor, process the milk, egg, and egg white until well mixed but stop short of creating foam. Add the flour, sugar (if desired), and any spices you want to try and pulse until just mixed. The batter should be quite thin. Add more milk as necessary.

Heat a lightly greased medium skillet or crepe pan over medium heat. The pan is ready when a drop of water dropped in the pan dances on the surface. For each crepe, use 3 tablespoons of batter. Immediately swirl the pan gently to distribute the batter in a very thin layer. Cook the crepe until the surface appears dry, about 1 minute. Stack cooked crepes on a plate with wax paper between each to prevent sticking. Fill the crepes lightly with your favorite filling—I love applesauce or orange marmalade. Roll and enjoy.

Spinach Soufflé
(Serves 4)

> 1 large egg
> ⅓ cup low-fat milk
> ⅓ cup grated Parmesan cheese
> 1 teaspoon crushed garlic
> Salt and pepper to taste
> Two 10-ounce packages frozen leaf spinach, thawed

Preheat oven to 350°F. In a medium bowl whisk together the egg, milk, cheese, garlic, salt, and pepper. Fold in the spinach. Place in a small casserole dish. Bake for 20 minutes, or until lightly set.

Breakfast "Martini"
(Serves 1)

> 3 large frozen strawberries, almost thawed
> ½ cup frozen blueberries, almost thawed
> ½ cup of your favorite granola cereal
> 3 ounces low-fat vanilla pudding
> Fat-free whipped cream topping
> 1 maraschino cherry

In your favorite martini glass, layer your ingredients in ¼-inch-thick layers. Start with a single strawberry, then a layer of blueberries, then the granola, next the pudding. Repeat until the glass is full. Top with whipped cream, a sprinkle of granola, and the single, decorative cherry.

Julia's Bran Muffins
(Makes 2 to 2½ dozen muffins)

> 2½ cups whole wheat flour
> 4 teaspoons double-acting baking powder
> ½ cup wheat germ
> ½ cup flaxseed
> 1 teaspoon each of ground cinnamon and salt
> ½ cup butter
> ¼ cup vegetable shortening
> ½ cup sugar
> ½ cup Equal Sugar Lite
> ½ cup applesauce
> 2 eggs plus 1 egg white
> 2¼ cups skim milk
> 2¼ cups whole oats, uncooked
> 1 cup raisins, ½ cup walnuts, or ½ cup dried cranberries (optional)

Preheat oven to 375°F. Line large muffin pans with liners. In a small bowl, combine the flour, baking powder, wheat germ, flaxseed, cinnamon, and salt and set aside. Using an electric mixer, in a mixing bowl cream the butter, shortening, and sugars until light and fluffy. Add the eggs and beat until combined. Stir in the applesauce. Alternately beat in flour mixture, and milk, a little of each at a time, beating well after each addition. Stir in the oats and add more milk if mixture looks too thick. Add any of the optional ingredients. Fill each baking cup with an equal amount of batter about two-thirds full. Bake for 20 to 25 minutes or until muffins are lightly browned and a toothpick inserted in the center comes out dry. Remove muffins to a wire rack to cool.

Zucchini Bread
(Makes 2 loaves. Each loaf serves 12)

> 3 cups shredded zucchini
> 4 cups whole wheat flour
> 1¼ cup sugar
> ½ cup chopped walnuts
> ¼ cup brown sugar

5 teaspoons baking powder
1 tablespoon grated lemon rind
2 teaspoons pumpkin pie spice
½ teaspoon salt
1½ cups skim milk
2 large eggs, beaten
6 tablespoons vegetable oil
2 teaspoons pure vanilla extract

Preheat oven to 350°F. Spray two 8 × 4-inch loaf pans with Pam.

Dry the zucchini on paper towels. Mix the flour, 1 cup of the sugar, the walnuts, brown sugar, baking powder, lemon rind, pumpkin pie spice, and salt in a large mixing bowl. Form a crater in the center. Combine the milk, eggs, oil, and vanilla. Stir in the zucchini. Add the mixture to the flour, stirring until moistened. Divide the batter between loaf pans evenly. Sprinkle remaining sugar on top. Bake for 1 hour or until a wooden toothpick inserted in the center comes out clean. Cool for 5 minutes and remove from the pans. Cool completely on a wire rack.

 MIDDAY FUEL AND SALADS

Grilled Chicken Breast
(Serves 2)

½ teaspoon cumin
1 tablespoon fresh cilantro, chopped
½ tablespoon lime juice
pepper, to taste
2 chicken breasts

Mix all ingredients in bowl. Marinate chicken for 1 hour. Grill or broil until tender (approximately 4 minutes on each side).

Fruity Jicama Salad
(Serves 5)

> 1 teaspoon grated orange rind
> ¼ cup fresh orange juice
> 2 tablespoons brown sugar
> ¾ teaspoon pumpkin pie spice
> 3 cups julienne-cut peeled jicama
> 1 ruby red grapefruit, peeled and sectioned
> 2 oranges, peeled and sliced crosswise
> 2 kiwifruit, peeled and sliced

Combine the orange rind, juice, sugar, and spice in a medium bowl and stir with a whisk. Add the jicama, grapefruit, orange, and kiwi, tossing gently. Serve with a grilled chicken breast for the perfect lunch.

Warm Pear Salad with Blue Cheese
(Serves 4)

> ¼ cup water
> 1 tablespoon sugar
> 1 tablespoon red wine vinegar
> ½ teaspoon beef bouillon granules
> 2 cups finely shredded red cabbage
> 1 cup chopped peeled pears (Anjou are my favorite)
> 2 cups baby spinach
> 4 teaspoons crumbled blue cheese

Combine the water, sugar, vinegar, and bouillon in a large skillet over high heat. Cover, reduce the heat, and simmer 1 minute. Add the cabbage to skillet and sauté for 2 minutes. Add pears and sauté 2 minutes or until pears are crisp-tender; remove from heat. Place ¼ cup of the baby spinach on each plate and divide the sauté mix among the plates. Garnish with the blue cheese. Serve with a piece of grilled fish—a perfect meal.

Tuna Fish–Stuffed Tomatoes
(Serves 2)

> 2 large tomatoes
> One 12-ounce can water-packed tuna
> 2 tablespoons sweet pickle relish
> 1 teaspoon pepper
> 2 egg whites, hard boiled and diced
> 2 tablespoons no-fat mayonnaise
> 2 tablespoons shredded low-fat Cheddar cheese

Cut off the top quarter of each tomato and scoop out the pulp, discarding tops and pulp. In a medium bowl mix the tuna, relish, pepper, eggs, and mayonnaise and spoon into the tomatoes. Top with the Cheddar. Broil until the cheese starts to bubble and turn slightly brown.

Hail Caesar
(Serves 2)

> 2 cups baby spinach leaves
> ½ cup cooked long-grain brown rice
> ½ cup cooked peas and pearl onions (buy frozen bag)
> 1 avocado, cubed
> 1 tablespoon balsamic vinegar
> 2 tablespoons low-fat Caesar dressing
> 2 grilled chicken breasts, sliced (see recipe on page 187)
> 2 teaspoons shredded Asiago or Parmesan cheese

This couldn't be any easier. Place the spinach in a bowl and add all the other ingredients. Stir until dressings are tossed evenly and serve.

Veggie Sandwich
(Serves 1)

> 1 tablespoon chive light cream cheese
> 2 slices dense fiber-filled bread
> ¼ cucumber, sliced thin
> 2 to 3 slices of tomato
> 1 to 2 sliced pepperoncini
> 1 sliced red onion
> Pile of bean sprouts
> 2 thinly sliced pieces of zucchini
> 1 slice mozzarella cheese

Spread the cream cheese on the bread and stack the remaining ingredients. Slice in half and serve. A nice glass of mint tea is the perfect addition to this great lunch.

Roast Beef Sandwich
(Serves 1)

> 2 slices hearty fiber-filled bread
> 5 ounces lean roast beef
> 1 slice low-fat Alpine Cheddar
> Romaine or red leaf lettuce
> 3 slices tomato
> Yellow onion slices to taste
> 1 teaspoon mayonnaise
> Country Dijon mustard to taste

Toast both pieces of bread lightly in a toaster oven, add beef and cheese, and toast lightly until the cheese starts to melt. Stack on all other ingredients and serve open-face style.

Summer salad
(Serves 6)

> ¼ cup raspberry vinegar
> 2 tablespoons honey
> 2 teaspoons olive oil
> ¼ cup seedless raspberry jam
> 8 cups raw spinach leaves
> 2 cups cantaloupe balls
> 1½ cups strawberries, halved
> 1 cup blackberries
> ¼ cup chopped macadamia nuts

Whisk the vinegar, honey, oil, and jam until mixed well. Combine the spinach and fruits in a bowl and toss with the dressing. Sprinkle with nuts and serve. Is there any salad when combined with a grilled chicken breast that isn't the perfect meal?

Ranch Slaw
(Serves 6)

> ⅓ cup sliced green onions
> One 10-ounce package angel hair slaw
> ⅓ cup fat-free ranch dressing
> One 11-ounce can mandarin oranges in water, drained
> 1 avocado, peeled and cut into small cubes

Combine onions and slaw in a large bowl. Add the dressing and toss to coat. Add the oranges and avocado. Toss gently. Serve immediately.

Wild Rice Oriental Salad
(Serves 8)

> 3 cups water
> ½ cup uncooked wild rice
> 1½ cups uncooked long-grain brown rice
> 1½ cups chopped red bell peppers
> 1 cup diagonally cut celery
> 1 cup frozen peas, thawed
> One 8-ounce can water chestnuts, drained and chopped
> ½ cup sliced green onions
> ⅓ cup thawed orange juice concentrate
> ¼ cup low-sodium soy sauce
> 1 tablespoon vegetable oil
> 1½ teaspoons lemon juice
> 1 tablespoon freshly grated ginger (time-consuming, but so good!)
> 2 cloves garlic, minced
> Lettuce leaves
> 2 tablespoons unsalted cashews

Bring the water to a boil in a large saucepan. Add the wild rice, cover, and reduce heat. Cook for 10 minutes and add brown rice. Cover and simmer 50 minutes, or until tender. Drain the rice mixture and transfer to a large bowl. Add the bell peppers, celery, peas, water chestnuts, and onions. Combine the orange juice with the soy sauce, oil, lemon juice, ginger, and garlic, pour over the rice, and toss well. Cover and chill for 2 hours. Arrange the lettuce leaves on plates and add the rice mixture. Sprinkle with cashews before serving. If you wish, add 1 cup cooked lentils for more protein. Then it is a stand-alone dish.

Tabbouleh
(Serves 5)

> 1½ cups uncooked bulgur or cracked wheat
> 1½ cups boiling water
> 3 teaspoons olive oil
> 1½ cups diced white onion
> Bunch of cilantro

5 stalks green onion
Bunch of parsley
1 cucumber, skinned, seeded, and diced
¼ cup slivered almonds, toasted
5 tablespoons lemon juice
1 tablespoon ground cumin
1½ teaspoons dried oregano
½ teaspoon salt
⅛ teaspoon ground allspice

Put the bulgur in boiling water, stir well, cover, and let stand for 30 minutes or until liquid is absorbed. Heat 1 teaspoon of the oil in a small skillet, add the onion, and sauté until tender. Add the onion to the bulgur. In a food processor finely chop the cilantro, green onion, and parsley. Put the bulgur mixture into a bowl, add the chopped mixture and the cucumber, and stir in the almonds, lemon juice, cumin, remaining olive oil, oregano, salt, and allspice. Chill until you serve it.

Black Bean Couscous
(Serves 2)

1 large orange
⅛ teaspoon salt
⅔ cup uncooked couscous
1 cup canned black beans, rinsed and drained
½ cup chopped red bell peppers
½ cup chopped green onions
2 tablespoons finely chopped parsley
1 tablespoon seasoned rice vinegar
1½ teaspoons vegetable oil
¼ teaspoon cumin

Grate enough orange rind to yield ¼ teaspoon, and set aside. Squeeze the juice from orange over a bowl, reserve ¼ cup juice, and set aside. Add water to the remaining juice to make 1 cup and add the salt. Bring the mixture to a boil in a medium saucepan, gradually stirring in the couscous. Remove from heat. Cover and let stand for 5 minutes. Stir and cool 5 more minutes. Stir in the rind, beans, peppers, onions, and parsley. Combine the reserved orange juice with the vinegar, oil, and cumin. Pour over the couscous mixture and toss well. Store in an airtight container in the refrigerator. Chill until served.

Fancy Tuna Salad
(Serves 6)

> 6 small red potatoes, scrubbed and cleaned (not peeled) and with top and bottom sliced off
> ¾ pound trimmed fresh green beans
> 3 hard-boiled eggs
> 4 cups torn romaine lettuce
> 4 cups trimmed watercress (about 1 bunch)
> Two 12-ounce cans tuna, packed in water
> 3 tomatoes, each cut into 6 wedges
> 1 green pepper, cut into strips
> ½ cup nicoise or Kalamata olives
> 2 teaspoons minced garlic
> 2 tablespoons capers
> Balsamic vinaigrette bottled dressing

Steam the potatoes, covered, for 3 minutes. Add green beans and steam, covered, for about 5 minutes or until crisp-tender. Cool. Discard 2 of the egg yolks, reserving 1, and quarter the whites lengthwise.

On a platter combine the lettuce and watercress. Arrange the tuna, fluffed with a fork, the potatoes, green beans, tomato, egg whites, and bell pepper over the greens. Top with crumbled yolk, olives, garlic, and capers. Drizzle with vinaigrette.

Variation: You can use fresh tuna. Drizzle it with lemon juice and black pepper, marinate it for 15 minutes, and prepare it on a grill or in a broiler. Cut the tuna in chunks to serve.

Hearty Five-Bean Soup
(Serves 8)

½ cup navy beans
½ cup turtle beans
½ cup pinto beans
3 quarts low-fat or no-fat chicken stock
1 medium onion, diced
4 celery stalks, diced
2 carrots, diced
½ cup lentils
½ cup split peas
2 tablespoons marjoram, fresh or dried
2 teaspoons kosher salt
½ teaspoon black pepper

Soak the navy, turtle, and pinto beans overnight in water. Drain the beans completely. In a large kettle bring the chicken stock to a boil. Reduce heat to a simmer. Add the onions, celery, and carrots. Cook for 45 minutes, or until the beans are three-quarters cooked. Add the lentils and split peas and cook for 30 more minutes, or until tender. Remove half of the bean mixture and puree in a blender. Return it to the kettle and stir in the seasonings.

Waldorf Chicken Salad
(Serves 2)

4 tablespoons plain fat-free yogurt
6 tablespoons fat-free mayonnaise
2 tablespoons raisins
2 tablespoons dried cranberries
½ cup diced celery
2 tablespoons chopped walnuts
2 chicken breasts, grilled and diced
6 cups peeled, cored, and diced red delicious apples
4 strawberries
2 sprigs fresh mint

In a bowl, combine yogurt, mayonnaise, raisins, cranberries, celery, and walnuts. Mix chicken and apples together. Pour the dressing over the apple-chicken mixture and gently toss. Place on 2 plates and garnish with strawberries and mint.

 EVENING FUEL

Grilled Beef Tenderloin with Couscous
(Serves 2)

> 4 cups cooked couscous (prepared with low-fat chicken stock)
> 1 cup diced tomato
> 1 cup peeled, diced seedless cucumber
> ½ cup fat-free tangerine mint dressing
> ¼ cup fresh chopped mint
> ¼ cup fresh chopped parsley
> 2 tablespoons lemon juice
> ½ tablespoon minced garlic
> 1 teaspoon cumin
> Salt and pepper to taste
> 5 ounces beef tenderloin, cut into 2 pieces

In a bowl, combine the couscous, tomato, cucumber, tangerine mint dressing, mint, parsley, lemon juice, garlic, cumin, salt, and pepper. Charbroil the beef tenderloin to desired doneness and serve with the couscous.

Pork Tenderloin with Ziti
(Serves 2)

> 8 ounces pork tenderloin
> ¼ cup fat-free Italian dressing
> ¾ cup fat-free mayonnaise
> ½ cup fat-free sour cream

2 tablespoons chopped fresh dill
½ cup chopped scallions
¼ cup roasted red peppers
2 tablespoons Dijon mustard
2 tablespoons sweet relish
10 ounces cooked ziti

Marinate the pork in the dressing for 30 minutes. Combine the mayonnaise, sour cream, dill, scallions, peppers, mustard, and relish, and mix gently with the pasta. Slice the pork into medallions and charbroil until done to taste. Serve with the cooked ziti.

Serve hot.

Halibut Steaks Cabo San Lucas
(Serves 2)

Two 8-ounce halibut steaks
2 tablespoons fat-free lime-cilantro dressing
2 portions angel hair pasta (whole wheat works great with this)
6 tomato slices
Juice from ½ large orange
Juice from 1 lemon
Juice from 1 lime
¼ cup white wine
4 teaspoons chopped cilantro
2 sprigs cilantro

Marinate the halibut in fat-free lime cilantro dressing for 15 minutes. Cook the pasta according to directions, drain, but do not rinse. Charbroil the halibut for 3 minutes per side. Do not overcook. Grill tomato slices. Heat the pasta in the orange, lemon, and lime juice with the white wine and chopped cilantro until hot. Place the pasta on a plate with the grilled tomato and top with the halibut. Garnish with cilantro sprigs.

Cashew-Crusted Orange Roughy
(Serves 2)

> 2 tablespoons ground cashews
> 1 tablespoon flour
> 2 tablespoons Italian bread crumbs
> Two 7-ounce orange roughy pieces
> 2 tablespoons each: fresh basil, oregano, and parsley
> Paprika to taste

Preheat oven to 350°F. In a shallow dish, combine the cashews, flour, and bread crumbs. Stir in the herbs and paprika, and mix well. Coat the fish with the mixture completely. Place in a baking pan, sprayed with Pam. Sprinkle lightly with paprika. Bake the fish for 12 to 15 minutes or until it is done. Serve with a spinach salad tossed with mandarin oranges and slivered almonds and mixed with poppy seed dressing for a perfect meal.

Ham with Penne and Snow Peas
(Serves 2)

> ¾ cup julienned red onions
> ¾ cup julienned yellow onions
> 2 tablespoons minced garlic
> 1 pound snow peas, julienned
> 1 red pepper, sliced into julienne
> ½ tablespoon olive oil
> 6 ounces 95 percent fat-free turkey ham, julienned
> 1 cup fat-free or low-fat chicken stock
> 1 tablespoon fresh chopped thyme
> 2 tablespoons fresh chopped basil
> 6 ounces cooked penne
> 2 tablespoons grated Romano cheese
> Chopped parsley for garnish

Sauté the onions, garlic, snow peas, and peppers in olive oil. Add the turkey ham and heat. Add the chicken stock, thyme, and basil. Bring to a boil and add the penne. Gently toss, heat completely, and remove from heat. Serve with grated Romano cheese and garnish with chopped parsley.

Miso Salmon
(Serves 4)

> 1 tablespoon red miso paste
> 1 teaspoon peanut oil
> 2 tablespoons freshly grated or finely chopped ginger
> 2 tablespoons soy sauce
> 1 tablespoon rice wine vinegar
> 1 tablespoon honey
> Four 6-ounce skinless salmon fillets
> 2 heads of bok choy, cut in half lengthwise
> 8 ounces shiitake mushrooms, cut in half
> 6 scallions, peeled and cut into 1-inch lengths
> Freshly ground pepper

In a small bowl, whisk together the miso, oil, ginger, and 1 tablespoon of the soy sauce. Add the vinegar and honey and stir well. Place the salmon fillets in a shallow dish and pour the miso mixture over them until they are well coated. Cover with plastic wrap and refrigerate for 1 hour. Grill the salmon until done; do not overcook. Steam the bok choy, mushrooms, and scallions for 3 to 4 minutes. Remove from the heat and season with pepper. Serve the salmon topped with the veggies and drizzle with the remaining soy sauce.

Summer Veggies with Chicken and Pasta
(Serves 4)

> Juice of ½ lemon
> 1 tablespoon olive oil
> 1 teaspoon honey
> 2 scallions, finely chopped
> 2 tablespoons roughly chopped tarragon
> 10 spears fresh asparagus
> 1 cup thickly sliced baby zucchini
> ¾ cup frozen peas and pearl onions
> 1 pound 2 ounces fresh fettuccine
> 12 cherry tomatoes, cut in half
> Freshly ground pepper
> 4 grilled chicken breasts (marinated in Italian dressing prior to grilling)
> 4 tablespoons fresh Romano cheese

Mix the lemon juice, olive oil, honey, scallions, and tarragon together. Prepare asparagus by breaking off the ends and carefully peeling the tips. Cut into 1-inch lengths. Cook the asparagus for 2 minutes in boiling water, remove with a slotted spoon, and quickly place in cold water. Add the zucchini to boiling water for 1 minute; remove, and quickly place in cold water. Add the peas and pearl onions to the boiling water and cook for 3 minutes; remove and add to cold water. Cook the fresh pasta in plenty of boiling water for 2 to 3 minutes. Drain the pasta, reserving ¼ cup of the cooking water. Return the pasta to the pan, add drained veggies and tomatoes, and toss well. Add the lemon dressing, reserved cooking water, and pepper to taste. Toss well. Add sliced grilled chicken breasts and toss. Garnish with the Romano cheese.

Pumpkin Risotto
(Serves 4)

> 1 pound pumpkin, peeled and cut into ½-inch dice
> 1 medium white onion, finely chopped
> 1 garlic clove, crushed
> Oil-water spray (prepared by using 7 parts water to 1 part olive oil or
>   canola oil)

Freshly ground pepper
1 cup uncooked risotto rice
Peel of ½ lemon
3 cups boiling vegetable stock
1 ounce finely grated Parmesan cheese

Preheat the oven to 400°F. Place the pumpkin, onion, and garlic in a nonstick ovenproof casserole dish. Spray lightly with the oil-water spray and season with pepper. Place in oven for 15 to 20 minutes, until golden and caramelized, turning regularly. Sprinkle the rice and lemon peel over the pumpkin and stir well. Pour in the boiling vegetable stock and stir well. Cover the dish with foil and return it to the oven for 25 to 30 minutes, or until the rice is tender and all the stock is absorbed. Stir in half of the Parmesan and garnish with the remaining cheese. Serve with a grilled turkey breast for the perfect fall meal.

Mango Salsa Snapper
(Serves 4)

¼ cup chopped green onion
1 green pepper, seeded and chopped
1 stalk celery, peeled and chopped
1 red chile, stem removed, chopped
1 tablespoon fresh thyme leaves
1 tablespoon marjoram leaves
⅓ cup chopped fresh parsley
Juice of 2 limes
4 garlic cloves, peeled
Freshly ground black pepper
Four 6-ounce skinless, snapper fillets, cleaned
Oil-water spray (prepared by using 7 parts water to 1 part olive oil or canola oil)

Mango Salsa
1 mango, peeled and cut into ½-inch dice
1 red onion, chopped
3 plum tomatoes, seeded and cut into ½-inch dice
1 garlic clove, crushed
Juice of 2 limes
3 tablespoons roughly chopped fresh mint leaves
1 teaspoon sugar

In blender, combine the green onion, pepper, celery, chile, thyme, marjoram, parsley, lime juice, garlic, and black pepper and process to a paste and place it in a shallow dish. Rub the snapper with paste on both sides. Cover with plastic wrap and marinate it at room temperature for at least 2 hours. Place all salsa ingredients in a small bowl and marinate for 30 minutes.

Preheat the oven to 450°F. Spray a nonstick baking tray with the oil-water spray, place snapper in it, and bake for 8 to 10 minutes until cooked. Serve with the salsa on top and brown rice.

Salmon Tortilla
(Serves 4)

1 teaspoon olive oil
1 small onion, finely chopped
One 14½-ounce can tomatoes, chopped and drained
1 tablespoon tomato paste
1 can anchovy fillets, drained and finely chopped
Four 8-inch soft wheat-flour tortillas
14 ounces smoked salmon, chopped into large pieces
2 scallions, shredded
2 tablespoons fresh dill, chopped, plus some sprigs for garnish
4 tablespoons low-fat mozzarella cheese, coarsely grated
2 tablespoons drained capers
Freshly ground pepper

Preheat the oven to 450°F. In a small pan, heat the oil, add the onion, and cook for 2 minutes over medium heat until softened. Add the tomatoes, tomato paste, and anchovies and cook for 6 to 8 minutes or until the mixture thickens to a pulpy consistency. Spread the tomato mixture evenly over the tortillas. Scatter the salmon on top, followed by the scallions, and chopped dill. Sprinkle the cheese over the top, place on large baking tray, and cook for 3 to 5 minutes or until cheese has melted. Sprinkle capers and dill sprigs over the top. Season to taste with pepper. Serve immediately.

Sesame Chicken
(Serves 4)

> 4 skinless chicken breasts, cut into cubes
> ½ cup water plus 1 tablespoon water
> ⅓ cup apple juice (not from concentrate; no sugar added)
> 2 tablespoons soy sauce
> 4 tablespoons sliced green onion
> 1 tablespoon ketchup
> 1 tablespoon dark brown sugar
> 2 garlic cloves, minced
> 1 teaspoon ground 3-color pepper, or to taste (red, green, and black)
> 1 teaspoon cornstarch
> 4 teaspoons toasted sesame seeds

Spray a 5-quart saucepan or Dutch oven with Pam and set over medium heat. Add the chicken and cook, turning, until chicken is browned on all sides; about 5 minutes. Transfer to a small platter and set aside. In small mixing bowl combine ½ cup water, the juice, soy sauce, onion, ketchup, sugar, and garlic. Season with the pepper, mixing well. Pour into the pan and cook over medium heat for 2 minutes, stirring constantly to scrape up any browned particles from the bottom. Reduce the heat to low. Add the chicken; cover, and cook until it is tender; about 20 minutes. Transfer the chicken to a platter, leaving liquid in the pot, and keep it warm. Dissolve the cornstarch in 1 tablespoon of water and add to the liquid. Cook, stirring frequently, until the sauce is thickened, about 4 minutes. Pour the sauce evenly over the chicken and sprinkle with sesame seeds.

Marinated Flank Steak
(Serves 4)

> ½ cup chopped shallots
> ⅓ cup red wine vinegar
> 3 tablespoons balsamic vinegar
> 2 teaspoons Montreal Steak (pepper) seasoning
> 1½ pounds flank steak, trimmed
> ¼ teaspoon salt

Combine the shallots and vinegars in a large Ziploc plastic bag and add 1 teaspoon pepper seasoning and the steak. Marinate in fridge 8 hours or overnight, turning occasionally.

Prepare a grill or preheat broiler. Remove the steak from the bag and discard the marinade. Sprinkle the steak with remaining pepper seasoning and the salt. Place the steak on grill rack or a broiler pan coated with Pam. Cook 6 minutes on each side or until desired degree of doneness. Cut steak diagonally across the grain into thin slices.

Italian Chicken with Chickpeas
(Serves 4)

> 1 pound chicken breast tenders
> ¼ teaspoon salt
> ¼ teaspoon pepper
> 1 tablespoon olive oil
> 1⅓ cups sliced white onion
> 1 cup green bell pepper strips
> 1 tablespoon minced garlic
> One 15½-ounce can chickpeas, drained
> One 14½-ounce can diced tomatoes, drained
> 1 tablespoon chopped basil
> 1 tablespoon chopped oregano

Sprinkle the chicken with salt and pepper. Heat the oil in a large non-stick skillet over medium-high heat. Add the chicken, and cook it for 2 minutes on each side or until browned. Add onion and bell pepper and sauté 4 minutes. Reduce the heat to medium. Add the garlic, chickpeas, tomatoes, basil, and oregano and cook for 8 minutes or until thoroughly heated.

Scallop Spaghetti
(Serves 4)

> 3 teaspoons olive oil
> 2 pounds sea scallops
> ½ teaspoon salt
> ½ teaspoon black pepper
> 2 tablespoons butter
> ½ cup minced green onions
> 1 tablespoon bottled minced garlic
> ⅔ cup dry white wine
> 2 tablespoons fresh lemon juice
> 4 servings fresh-cooked angel hair pasta
> 2 tablespoons finely chopped fresh parsley
> 1 lemon, thinly sliced for garnish

Heat the oil in a large nonstick skillet over medium-high heat. Sprinkle the scallops with salt and pepper. Add the scallops to the pan and sauté them for 2 minutes on each side. Remove the scallops from pan and keep them warm wrapped in aluminum foil. Add the butter to pan with the green onions and garlic and sauté for 30 seconds. Add the wine and juice and cook 1 minute. Return the scallops to the pan and toss to coat. Remove from the heat. Place scallops on top of the pasta, spoon on remaining sauce, and garnish with parsley and lemon.

Recommended Products and Resources

Throughout this book you have seen references to a few products; below you can find more information about them and/or where to learn more. These products are my personal preferences and the ones that I use on a daily basis. Many of my readers use the same products, and I believe that they do play an essential role in my patients' success and in my ongoing preventative health measures and maintaining my 130-pound weight loss. If you have any questions you can reach me for more information.

Motivational support tools: www.ViceBustingDiet.com. You can get the complete 26-week LifeChanger journal, *Getting Started* video, *Basic Exercise* video, and numerous audios AND weekly teleconferences and more—the perfect complement to *The Vice-Busting Diet*.

Eating plans, community support, and expert interaction: www.ediets.com/JuliaHavey. Here you can join me on my support board, "Take It Off w/ Julia," take part in live eDiets.com monthly chats with me as well as other outstanding experts, interact with a community of millions of people just like you, and choose from a variety of individualized eating plans from a team of superior nutritionists.

Whole food nutrition: Juice Plus+®: There are many products to choose from when making the decision about what to eat. I recommend that you do your research thoroughly and I think it will be clear that there is nothing better than Juice Plus+® for you, your family, and anyone whose health you care about. This is a MUST if you want to be optimally healthy.

Pedometers: www.Walk4Life.com. They make a good product and stand behind it with a one-year warranty—that speaks volumes to me about how well it works. Buy theirs, or a different one, but either way, get a pedometer today.

Home exercise equipment: www.OctaneFitness.com. The BEST at-home piece of cardiovascular equipment on the market. This is not only my personal opinion but it is also shared by everyone I know who has one.

Exercise videos and weighted bars: For great home workouts visit www.bodybars.com: one bar, infinite workouts. And coming in late 2006 watch for Julia and Patrick's Total Body Bar home exercise DVD.

www.askdrpat.com: For information from Dr. Patrick Havey on how to increase your energy, lower your cholesterol, and raise your fitness level.

You can find direct links to these and other helpful products at www.JuliaHavey.com. It is my goal to continue to bring you information about health must-haves on this journey, so check in with me and arm yourself with the essentials.

❧ Index

About the Authors

JULIA GRIGGS HAVEY

I was once a 290-pound unhappy single mother. I turned my life around, losing 130 pounds in the process. I have gone on to help millions of people to improve their lives and health as the "Master Motivator" to 14 million readers at eDiets.com. I am proud to be the author of the bestselling *Awaken the Diet Within*, which *USA Today* called a "must-read" book. I have appeared on QVC, *The Sally Jessy Raphael Show*, and *The Wayne Brady Show*, have been featured in *Glamour*, *Woman's World*, *First for Women*, and have been on dozens of radio stations across the nation. Two of my success-story women have appeared on the *cover* of *Woman's World*. My honest and common-sense approach has turned the dieting world upside down and is a voice of reason in the sea of fads and fake promises. I think the fact that I was once obese lets readers relate to me and realize that I am not offering them a theory of what *might* work, but rather showing them what *did* work—for me personally as well as thousands of others.

I am a former Mrs. Missouri, happily married to Dr. J. Patrick Havey, and together we are raising two children: daughter, Taylor, the emerging country-singing sensation and stunning beauty, and son, Clark, the hilarious Magician Musician and athletic ball of energy.

I love taking body-pump and kickboxing classes, doing weight lifting, and using my elliptical machine every day (yes, every day). I also enjoy traveling, reading, skiing, and playing games and cards.

J. PATRICK HAVEY, D.C.

I am the president of the Health & Wellness Institute, PC. I received my doctoral training at Logan College of Chiropractic in St. Louis, Missouri. In practice, I have seen firsthand the damage that obesity has caused to many patients—spinal injuries, arthritis, joint problems, and just an overall compromise in health. During my time in practice, I became interested in helping to solve this epidemic. I have made a mission of bringing real answers and practical solutions to individuals so that they can improve their health, and ultimately the health of our nation. I believe that a holistic approach is the best approach—considering all aspects and influences on the body and mind—for optimal results. I collaborated with Julia on *Awaken the Diet Within* and the very popular LifeChanger Program, both of which have been tremendously successful for readers, allowing them to realize results that had eluded them for years. I was happy to help contribute to *The Vice-Busting Diet* and believe it is the answer to the obesity epidemic.

I actively participate in many sports, enjoy weight training, and have taken part in several mini-triathlons. Julia is my loving wife, partner, and best friend.